Understanding Pharmacology

Susan M. Turley, CMT
RN, BSN, MA (Educ.)

PRENTICE HALL CAREER & TECHNOLOGY
Englewood Cliffs, New Jersey 07632

Cover design: *Mike Fender*
Prepress buyer: *Ilene Levy*
Manufacturing buyer: *Ed O'Dougherty*
Acquisitions editor: *Mark Hartman*
Editorial Assistant: *Louise Fullam*
Marketing Manager: *Ann Elizabeth Hendrix*

©1991 by Prentice Hall Career & Technology
Prentice-Hall, Inc.
A Paramount Communications Company
Englewood Cliffs, New Jersey 07632

Printed in the United States of America

10 9 8 7 6 5 4 3 2

PREVIOUSLY PUBLISHED BY:
HEALTH PROFESSIONS INSTITUTE, P.O. BOX 801, MODESTO, CA 95353

ISBN 0-13-126830-9

PRENTICE-HALL INTERNATIONAL (UK) LIMITED, London
PRENTICE-HALL OF AUSTRALIA PTY. LIMITED, Sydney
PRENTICE-HALL CANADA INC., Toronto
PRENTICE-HALL HISPANOAMERICANA, S.A., Mexico
PRENTICE-HALL OF INDIA PRIVATE LIMITED, New Delhi
PRENTICE-HALL OF JAPAN, INC., Tokyo
SIMON & SCHUSTER ASIA PTE. LTD., Singapore
EDITORA PRENTICE-HALL DO BRASIL, LTDA., Rio de Janeiro

To Al and Daniel

Preface

Pharmacology is a fascinating and multifaceted discipline which impacts not only on our professional careers but on our personal lives as well. From our role as members of the healthcare team to that of consumers, pharmacology plays a part in our lives.

The study of pharmacology covers a broad spectrum of diverse yet interrelated topics, such as botany, molecular chemistry, research, clinical observation, toxicology, legislation, and patient education.

There is an excitement inherent in its study that stretches from understanding the historical use of herbs and plant extracts, to seeing painstaking research produce both unusable products as well as life-saving discoveries, to finally viewing the future with its nearly limitless potential for medical discovery.

The purpose of this book is to serve as a guide to the reader in the study of pharmacology. The road of pharmacology is paved with extensive and often unrecognized research on the part of thousands of doctors and scientists around the world, built layer by layer on previous discoveries, with hard work, astute observation and, not infrequently, sudden insights and divinely appointed coincidences. This road is constantly being built anew with each drug discovery.

It is not the purpose of this book to be an exhaustive source of all drugs in current usage, to list drug dosages and side effects, or to instruct in the prescribing of medication; rather it is to provide a framework of thinking for healthcare professionals, laying a foundation of knowledge about drug theory and treatment, so that the road of pharmacology that stretches ahead will become both familiar and useful to the reader, to be traveled frequently in the future.

Acknowledgments

I am grateful to Sally C. Pitman, CMT, MA; Linda C. Campbell, CMT; Vera Pyle, CMT; and the staff of Health Professions Institute for their unfailing encouragement and faith in this project, and most particularly to John H. Dirckx, M.D., for his insightful comments and expertise in medical language.

Contents

Figures

Foreword

The classical Greek word *pharmakon,* on which the term *pharmacology* is based, had three related meanings: "charm," "poison," and "remedy." These variant senses of the word spotlight important aspects of the history of pharmacology.

In the prescientific age, issues of cause-and-effect were frequently assumed without experimental proof. What we now call superstition and magic took the place of more rational modes of thought and action. Primitive healers used natural substances of animal, vegetable, and mineral origin with boundless confidence in their power to cure, even though objective evidence of their efficacy was lacking. And we can be sure that many cures took place through the power of suggestion, a potent force still recognized today as the "placebo effect."

But if some patients recovered after dosing with crude, prehistoric remedies, others were killed outright. It cannot have escaped the early medicine men—or their patients—that some "medicines" were more useful for getting rid of enemies (or inconvenient friends) than for treating the sick. Hence the second meaning of *pharmakon.* Even today the toxicity of drugs is a major problem, for some of our most effective ones also have the narrowest margins of safety.

Only after centuries of observation and experimentation has medical science achieved an understanding of the ways drugs work and a sound basis for their safe and effective use. The third sense of *pharmakon,* a sense hedged about with a great deal of wishful thinking in primitive times, has thus largely been realized today. And yet in many ways we have only scratched the surface.

Many medicines achieve their effects not by neatly eliminating or neutralizing the source of symptoms but by inducing abnormalities in body chemistry or function that tend to offset the abnormalities caused by disease. Except for a few naturally occurring enzymes, hormones, vitamins, and minerals, most substances administered as medicines are foreign to the body and therefore capable of causing annoying side effects and allergic reactions. Clearly this state of affairs leaves much to be desired and presents a continuing challenge to pharmacologic chemists and clinical researchers.

The fact that we don't have a single perfect drug, much less a panacea or cure-all, accounts for the staggering multitude and diversity of imperfect ones in current use. The great number and variety of drugs are apt to prove daunting at first sight to the paraprofessional who undertakes the study of medical therapeutics.

I am sometimes asked, "How can you possibly remember all those drugs?" The answer is simple. I can't, and neither can anyone else. The typical practicing physician has a working knowledge of just one or two drugs in each pharmacologic class—perhaps more in classes pertaining to his specialty, perhaps none in classes he never has occasion to prescribe. Once a physician is fully familiar with the characteristics, indications, side effects, and dosage of one drug in a pharmacologic class, similar information about all the others in the same class would be excess baggage.

Just as the range of useful information for the practicing physician doesn't include the whole field of pharmacology, medical transcriptionists, medical records technicians, insurance clerks, and others involved in handling medical reports don't need to memorize huge masses of information or endless lists of drugs. What they need is a general understanding of how various kinds of drugs work, their potentials and limitations, some of the reasons for their number and diversity, and the rationale behind their bewildering and often tongue-twisting names.

That is the kind of mental data base that *Understanding Pharmacology* will give you. The author, drawing on her diversified background in nursing, medical transcription, and teaching, has produced a clear, well-organized, stimulating textbook that takes the student step-by-step through the whole subject of pharmacology without going into needless complexities or irrelevant details. The facts are accurate and up-to-date and their logical connections are presented with clarity and simplicity. Historical sidelights and pertinent illustrations keep the interest level high. A concise glossary at the end of the book gives capsule information about hundreds of current drugs.

Understanding Pharmacology is not only a superb introductory textbook but a reference work that you will consult often and with profit.

John H. Dirckx, M.D.

1

Introduction to Pharmacology

Pharmacology is the study of drugs and their interactions with living organisms. The term *pharmacology* comes from the Greek words *pharmakon* meaning *medicine* and the suffix *-ology* meaning *the study of.* Pharmacology is concerned with the nature of drugs and medications, their actions in the body, drug dosages, and side effects.

Pharmacology is a general term. Other more specific terms related to the study of drugs include:

> pharmacodynamics—how drugs produce their effects
> pharmacokinetics—mathematical descriptions of drug response based on time and dose
> molecular pharmacology—the chemical structure of drugs at a molecular level
> toxicology—the study of toxic or poisonous effects of drugs

The term *drug* is derived from the Dutch word *droog* which means *dry* and refers to the use of dried herbs and plants as the first medicines. The Latin word for drug is *medicina* from which we derive *medicine.*

In the first eleven chapters of this book, we will discuss the following topics:

> An overview of the history of drugs
> Drug legislation
> Drug design and manufacturing
> Drug forms and routes of administration
> Steps in the drug cycle
> Effects of drugs
> Drug terminology
> Systems of drug measurement
> The drug prescription

All of these subjects serve as introductory material to lay a strong foundation of basic knowledge upon which to build expertise in specific drugs. The chapters which follow then introduce commonly prescribed drugs according to body system to facilitate learning. The material presented in each chapter will include brief historical notes, details of pharmaceutical action of various drugs, and clinical notes on current therapeutic applications.

REVIEW QUESTIONS

1. Describe the linguistic origins of the following words:
   pharmacology
   medicine/medication
   drug

2. A knowledge of drug forms, routes of administration, drug effects, and drug measurement is an essential foundation for understanding the action and use of specific drugs. True or False?

2

The History of Drugs: An Overview

Pharmacology is one of the oldest branches of medicine. Ancient peoples such as the Sumerians and Egyptians recorded the use of drugs on clay tablets and papyrus as early as 2000 B.C. At that time, diseases were treated with frog's bile, sour milk, lizard's blood, pig's teeth, spider's web, hippopotamus oil, and toad's eyelids. The ancient Egyptians applied moldy bread to abrasions, a practice which may have had some therapeutic basis as, many centuries later, penicillin was extracted from a mold.

Ancient drug preparations could contain many ingredients prepared according to standard recipes which involved drying, crushing, and combining a variety of plants or organic substances. The symbol *Rx,* which comes from the Latin word *recipe,* meaning *take,* indicates a *prescription,* the combining of ingredients to form a drug.

The use of some ingredients was based on medical lore, some on superstition. Some ingredients had therapeutic value, others were worthless, and some ingredients were quite harmful.

Because little was known about even the most fundamental physical and chemical processes of the body, the therapeutic use of drugs was a matter of much guessing. Medieval physicians prescribed opium and gold as well as herbs. In the 1600s, patients were advised to eat soap to cure hematuria and to drink mercury in beer to cure intestinal worms.

However, a number of drugs, based on old prescriptions, are still in use today.

The medicinal use of the foxglove plant (*Digitalis lanata*) has been noted in thirteenth century writings. A derivative, digoxin (Lanoxin), is still the drug of choice in treating congestive heart failure. See Figure 2-1.

The belladonna plant was the original source of two drugs which are still in use today—atropine and scopolamine. Belladonna means *beautiful lady* in Italian. "Sixteenth century Italian women . . . squeezed the berries of these plants into their eyes to widen and brighten them." (Michael C. Gerald, *Pharmacology: An Introduction to Drugs,* 2nd ed. [Englewood Cliffs, N.J.: Prentice-Hall, 1981], p. 149.)

Atropine is still used to dilate the pupil in patients with inflammatory conditions of the iris. Scopolamine is used for motion sickness, but has a side effect of blurred vision from paralysis of the muscles of accommodation around the pupil.

3

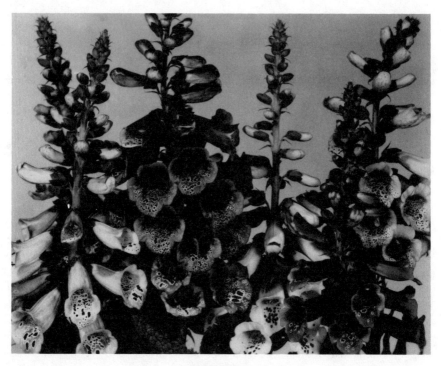

FIGURE 2-1

Digitalis lanata, or foxglove plant, the original source of the cardiac drug digitalis. Photo courtesy of W. Atlee Burpee Company, Warminster, PA.

Colchicine, a drug used in the treatment of gout, was used for that same purpose in the sixth century. It was originally derived from the meadow saffron flower known as *Colchicum autumnale.*

The over-the-counter bronchodilator ephedrine (Primatene, Bronkaid) is present in the leaves of the bushy shrub (species name, *Ephedra*) which were burned by the ancient Chinese to treat respiratory ailments.

DID YOU KNOW? Herbs have been a part of all cultures for centuries and mentioned frequently in literature. Henbane, a very toxic herb, was supposed to have been the poison which Claudius used to kill his brother, Hamlet's father. Dried henbane leaf is related to the belladonna plant, the original source of the modern-day drugs atropine and scopolamine (Transderm-Scōp). "Henbane should not be confused with wolfsbane. Students of literature know wolfsbane to be useful as a vampire repellant (Dracula, 1897); however, we should point out that double-blind studies demonstrating the effectiveness of this plant have not as yet been conducted." (Gerald, p. 149.)

In addition, many of the gums, oils, and bases in which drugs are carried come from animal and plant sources. The drug Accutane, which is used for severe cystic acne, contains beeswax and soybean oil in its capsule. Other drugs in capsules contain sesame seed oil or olive oil. Lanolin, a common ingredient of topical skin drugs, is obtained from the purified fat of processed sheep's wool.

The following table lists the original sources of some common modern drugs.

Plant, Animal, Mineral Source	Modern Drug
foxglove (*Digitalis lanata*)	digoxin (Lanoxin)
rose hips	vitamin C
belladonna	atropine
	scopolamine (Transderm-Scōp)
willow bark	aspirin
cinchona bark	quinine
opium poppy	morphine
vinca (periwinkle)	vincristine (Oncovin)
snakeroot (*Rauwolfia serpentina*)	reserpine (Serpasil)
mold	penicillin
beef or pork pancreas	insulin
minerals	iron, calcium

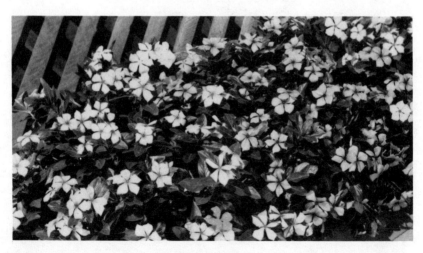

FIGURE 2-2
Vinca (periwinkle), the original source of the chemotherapy drugs vinblastine (Velban) and vincristine (Oncovin). Photo courtesy of W. Atlee Burpee Company, Warminster, PA.

It was not until the 1800s that chemists developed techniques to extract and isolate pure substances from crude drug preparations. The isolation of morphine in 1806 by a German pharmacist marked the beginning of modern drug treatment based on chemically pure ingredients.

In the early 1900s, extraction and preparation of drugs was still a time-consuming process which involved test tubes, filters, and bunsen burners. Pharmacists at that time had daily duties of preparing drugs from prescriptions. They actually made milk of magnesia, paregoric, and syrup bases for liquid medicines. In addition, they hand-rolled cocoa butter suppositories. They measured drugs in minims, drams, ounces, grains, and scruples.

Many drugs are now completely synthetic rather than derived from natural sources. Others have undergone chemical modification and molecular restructuring to create new drugs which possess superior pharmaceutical action. In addition, the pharmacist prepares medications, dispenses them, and provides patient information.

The following table briefly notes some major pharmaceutical milestones since the 1800s.

1806	Morphine isolated from crude opium.
1899	Aspirin introduced.
1908	Sulfanilamide introduced as the first antibacterial agent.
1912	Phenobarbital introduced for epilepsy.
1913	Vitamins A and B discovered.
1922	Insulin isolated.
1938	Dilantin introduced for epilepsy.
1941	Penicillin introduced.
1946	Benadryl introduced (first antihistamine).
1948	Cortisone introduced (first corticosteroid).
1952	Thorazine introduced for psychosis.
1954	Meprobamate introduced for neurosis.
1957	Librium introduced for neurosis.
1958	Haldol introduced for psychosis.
1967	Inderal introduced for arrhythmias (first beta blocker).
1970	Levodopa introduced for Parkinson disease.
1977	Tagamet introduced for peptic ulcers.
1981	Verapamil introduced for arrhythmias (first calcium channel blocker).
1982	Human insulin introduced (first drug made using recombinant DNA technology).
1986	Orthoclone OKT3 (first monoclonal antibody).

REVIEW QUESTIONS

1. Give the meaning of and describe the linguistic origins of the symbol *Rx*.

2. Give the name of a medication in current usage which originated from the natural sources listed below.

Natural Source	*Medication*
foxglove plant	
sheep's wool	
rose hips	
mold	
beef pancreas	
periwinkle	

3. In what decade was each of the following drugs/drug technologies first introduced? Circle the correct answer.

insulin	1890s	1900s	1910s	1920s	1930s	1940s
penicillin	1890s	1900s	1910s	1920s	1930s	1940s
aspirin	1890s	1900s	1910s	1920s	1930s	1940s
cortisone	1890s	1900s	1910s	1920s	1930s	1940s
Vitamin A	1890s	1900s	1910s	1920s	1930s	1940s
Tagamet	1940s	1950s	1960s	1970s	1980s	1990s
Librium	1940s	1950s	1960s	1970s	1980s	1990s
recombinant DNA	1940s	1950s	1960s	1970s	1980s	1990s
Inderal	1940s	1950s	1960s	1970s	1980s	1990s

3

Drug Legislation

From the early history of pharmacology, most physicians attempted to treat patients accurately based on the little scientific knowledge available to them. As early as 2100 B.C., the Code of Hammurabi gave severe penalties for malpractice.

Throughout medical history many ineffective and even dangerous medicines have been prescribed. During the 1700s and 1800s **patent medicines** with such names as Warner's Safe Cure for Diabetes, Dr. Shreve's Anti-Gallstone Remedy, and Anti-Morbific Great Liver and Kidney Medicine were commonly sold without regulation and accompanied by extravagant claims of cures. These medicines often contained the addicting drugs opium or morphine without their presence being listed on the label. Mrs. Winslow's Syrup for infants' teething pain contained morphine. Ayer's Cherry Pectoral for respiratory ailments contained cherry flavoring and heroin.

> Thomas Beecham (1820-1907), an English manufacturer of patent drugs, had this advertisement printed in hymnbooks:
>> Hark the herald angels sing
>> Beecham's pills are just the thing.
>> Peace on earth and mercy mild
>> Two for man and one for child.
>
> Marian Ringo, *Nobody Said It Better: 2700 Wise and Witty Quotations About Famous People* (Rand McNally, 1980).

Warnings against misuse, addiction, or side effects did not exist. One drug prescribed for respiratory ailments, hydrocyanic acid, caused many deaths. (This poison, which as a gas contains cyanide, is used for legal executions.) "Let the buyer beware" was the prevailing dictum.

The Origins of Drug Laws

Laws were passed in the 1900s to protect the public from unscrupulous sellers as well as from worthless or actually harmful medicines then on the market. The manufacturers of patent medicines strongly opposed drug laws, but public outrage resulted in the passage of the first federal drug law in 1906. This law required the labeling of drugs to prevent substituting ingredients or mislabeling. It also stated that only drugs listed in the United States Pharmacopeia or National Formulary could be prescribed. However, many worthless patent medicines remained on the market because the burden of proof lay with the government to show fraud on the part of the seller.

Sulfonamide, an early antibacterial agent, was widely used in the United States in 1937. After an extensive advertising campaign aimed at physicians, a Tennessee company marketed a form of this drug in a raspberry-flavored base called "Elixir of Sulfonamide." It had been tested by the manufacturer for flavor and fragrance but not for safety. Elixirs are made from a sweetened alcohol base, but in this drug the base used was not alcohol but an industrial strength liquid solvent. A number of children died after having been given less than one ounce of this drug, and over 350 people were poisoned. At that time, a drug manufacturer did not need FDA approval before marketing a drug. In 1938, Congress passed the **Food, Drug, and Cosmetic Act** which previously had lacked the support it needed to pass. As a result, the government no longer needed proof of fraud to stop the sale of drugs. It could seize products suspected of being toxic. Secondly, the burden of proof was shifted to the drug manufacturers, who were required to provide data based on scientific experiments to show that their product was safe before they were allowed to market it. It became the job of the **Food and Drug Administration (FDA)** to review these data and evaluate the safety of drugs.

In the late 1950s, the drug thalidomide was developed in West Germany and used extensively to treat morning sickness early in pregnancy. The FDA refused to approve it for use in the United States without further studies. Before these additional studies by the manufacturer could be completed, evidence against the safety of the drug began to accumulate. Over 8000 deformed babies were born in Europe with deformed limbs ("seal limbs" or phocomelia). This tragedy resulted in the 1962 amendment to the 1938 Food, Drug, and Cosmetic Act which tightened control on existing prescription drugs and new drugs. It required that drugs be shown to be both safe and effective before being marketed. It also required manufacturers to report adverse side effects from new drugs. Since that time, many drugs have been removed from the market because of a lack of safety or because of unproved effectiveness.

It should be noted, however, that no drug is entirely safe and without potential side effects and risks. Even one of the oldest and most widely used over-the-counter drugs—aspirin—can cause serious side effects of gastric ulcer and bleeding.

The FDA can also remove a drug from the market even after it has been approved if unforeseen adverse side effects become apparent. In 1982 Oraflex was hailed as a breakthrough drug in the treatment of arthritis. Within three months, 500,000 prescriptions had been written for it. This nonsteroidal anti-inflammatory drug (NSAID) needed to be taken only once daily (due to its long half-life which was 25 to 32 hours in adults). However, within two months the deaths of a number of elderly patients on Oraflex were reported to the FDA. It was found that in these patients, the half-life of the drug could increase dramatically to as long as 100 hours (due to slower metabolism and excretion in the elderly), producing toxic symptoms and death. The Oraflex label did not clearly state the need to reduce dosages in elderly patients. This drug was removed from the market by the FDA and, due to adverse publicity, the manufacturer chose not to relabel the drug but to discontinue its manufacture.

While the FDA has prevented many unsafe drugs from reaching consumers and has removed many dangerous or worthless drugs from the market, critics point to a time lag in approving some important new drugs. Historically, many new drugs have been available in other countries for some time before receiving clearance by the FDA for use in the United States. Inderal, a widely used drug for hypertension and arrhythmias, was available in Europe for nearly ten years before it was approved for use in the United States in 1967.

Legislation Concerning Schedule Drugs

Drugs of abuse were first regulated by the Harrison Narcotics Act of 1914. It was replaced by the **Controlled Substances Act of 1970** which established the **Drug Enforcement Administration (DEA)** to regulate the manufacturing and dispensing of dangerous and potentially abused drugs. This law divided potentially addictive prescription drugs on the market into five categories or schedules based on their potential for causing **physical or psychological dependence.** These drugs are known as **schedule drugs** or **controlled substances.**

Schedule I
    High potential for abuse
    No current medical usage
    Examples: PCP, heroin, LSD
Schedule II
    High potential for abuse
    Current medical applications
    Severe physical and psychological dependence may result.
    Examples: Percodan, Demerol, morphine, codeine
Schedule III
    Some potential for abuse
    Current medical applications
    Moderate physical and psychological dependence may result.
    Examples: Tylenol With Codeine, paregoric
Schedule IV
    Low potential for abuse
    Current medical applications
    Limited to moderate physical and psychological dependence
      may result.
    Examples: Darvon, Librium, Valium, phenobarbital
Schedule V
    Limited potential for abuse
    Current medical applications
    Examples: Lomotil, cough syrups with codeine
      (Tussi-Organidin)

Every physician (and dentist and pharmacy) must register each year with the Drug Enforcement Administration (DEA) and be issued a DEA number in order to prescribe or dispense any schedule (controlled) drug. The physician's DEA number must be clearly written on any prescription for these drugs.

The label and packaging for a controlled substance and all of its advertisements must clearly show the drug's assigned schedule. This is written to the right of the drug name in the following way.

FIGURE 3-1
Symbol for a Schedule IV drug
The large "C" stands for "controlled substance." The number written inside (always a Roman numeral) indicates the assigned schedule number. With this symbol, it is important to remember that a "C" with the Roman numeral IV inside it does not denote that the drug is to be given I.V. but that it is a Schedule IV (four) controlled substance.

Other Drug Legislation

In 1983 the **Orphan Drug Act** was passed. Its purpose was to facilitate the development of new drugs to treat rare diseases. Normally, pharmaceutical companies are reluctant to spend the large amounts of time and money needed for research and testing of a drug if it has a limited market. The Orphan Drug Act provides tax credits for the manufacturer and simplifies the process of obtaining FDA approval for these new drugs for rare diseases.

Prescription and Over-the-Counter Drugs

Prescription drugs, both schedule and nonschedule, are defined as those drugs which are not safe to use except under professional medical supervision and which can only be prescribed by a physician or dentist. They are always identified on the label with the inscription: "Caution: Federal law prohibits dispensing without prescription."

In addition to prescription drugs, the FDA also regulates **over-the-counter (OTC)** drugs. An OTC drug is defined as one which is generally considered safe for consumers to use if the label directions and warnings are properly followed.

REVIEW QUESTIONS

1. Patent medicines frequently contained addictive ingredients not listed on the label. Name two such ingredients.
2. No drug is entirely safe and without potential side effects and risks. True or False?
3. What federal agency is empowered to review data on a drug's safety and clinical effectiveness and approve drugs for marketing?
4. You are writing an article criticizing the time lag in the United States for approval of new drugs already in clinical use in other countries. What example might you give to support your position?
5. You are writing an article, in rebuttal to the article mentioned above, defending the time lag as based on appropriate medical caution. What example might you give to support your position?
6. Describe how the Controlled Substances Act of 1970 categorized drugs of potential abuse and how physicians are affected by this legislation.
7. What is the meaning of the symbol in Fig. 3-1?
8. What is the purpose of the 1983 Orphan Drug Act?

4

Drug Design, Testing, Manufacturing, and Marketing

The development, testing, manufacturing, and eventual marketing of any particular drug is a time-consuming and expensive process. In the early 1900s, Paul Ehrlich, a German chemist, tested 605 separate arsenic compounds before finding the first drug known to cure syphilis, nicknamed "the magic bullet." Today, a pharmaceutical company may evaluate thousands of different chemicals before finding one which moves successfully through all phases of testing and is finally approved by the FDA for release and marketing. In this chapter, we will trace the steps from newly discovered or designed chemical to final FDA approval and clinical use of a drug.

Drug Names

From the moment of its discovery or design, every drug has a **chemical name** which describes its molecular structure and distinguishes it from all other drugs. The pharmaceutical company, together with a special organization known as the United States Adopted Names Council, then determines a second name for the drug, its **generic name.** When the FDA gives final approval for marketing, then the manufacturer alone selects a third name known as the **trade name** or **brand name,** which is a registered trademark. Only the original manufacturer has the right to advertise and market the drug under that trade name.

Spelling of Drug Names

The accurate spelling of drug names is critical. Throughout this text, tips will be given to assist in accurate spelling of drug names.

The spelling of some generic groups of drugs may be similar to reflect their chemical similarity. All of the following drugs are members of the benzodiazepine classification, used to treat anxiety.

Example: diazepam (Valium)
lorazepam (Ativan)
halazepam (Paxipam)
oxazepam (Serax)
prazepam (Centrax)

13

In general, the particular spelling of a brand name drug is proposed by the manufacturer for one of several reasons:

- To indicate the disease process being treated.
  Example: Azmacort, a drug used to treat asthma.
  Rythmol, a drug used to treat cardiac arrhythmias.
- To simplify the generic name while retaining its phonetic sound.
  Example: The generic drug pseudoephedrine is named Sudafed.
  The generic drug haloperidol is named Haldol.
  The generic drug ciprofloxacin is named Cipro.
- To indicate the source of a drug.
  Example: Premarin, a drug obtained from **preg**nant **mar**es' **urine**.
- To indicate the action of the drug.
  Example: Elavil, a drug used to elevate depressed mood.
  Asendin, a drug used to help patients ascend from depression.
- To indicate several drugs in combination.
  Example: The trade name drugs Serpasil, Apresoline, and Esidrix are combined into the new trade name drug, Ser-Ap-Es.
- To indicate how often the drug is to be taken.
  Example: Spectrobid, taken b.i.d. (twice a day; b.i.d. is an abbreviation for the Latin words *bis in die)*.
- To indicate the duration of drug action.
  Example: Slow-K, slow release potassium supplement.
- To indicate the strength of a drug.
  Example: Bactrim DS, a double-strength dose.
  Tavist-1, 1 mg tablets.
- To indicate the amount of active ingredients.
  Example: Tylenol No. 3 contains 30 mg of codeine.
  Tylenol No. 2 contains 15 mg of codeine.
- To reflect the manufacturer's identity.
  Example: Wyeth-Ayerst pharmaceutical company manufacturers Wycillin, Wygesic, Wytensin, Wydase, and Wyamycin E.

Some brand name drugs are particularly difficult to spell because drug manufacturers are not held to any particular linguistic standards. As noted above, Rythmol is used to treat cardiac arrhythmias, and yet the initial *h* found in the word *rhythm* has been deleted. Asendin is used to treat depression and yet the *c* found in *ascending* has been removed.

Drug Design

New drugs are discovered in one of two different ways.

1. A totally new chemical substance may be discovered in the environment, e.g., in soil samples, plants, and marine animals. Thousands of soil samples have been evaluated for evidence of antibiotic activity. Many new antibiotics have been discovered in this way. The fungus from which the cephalosporin antibiotics are

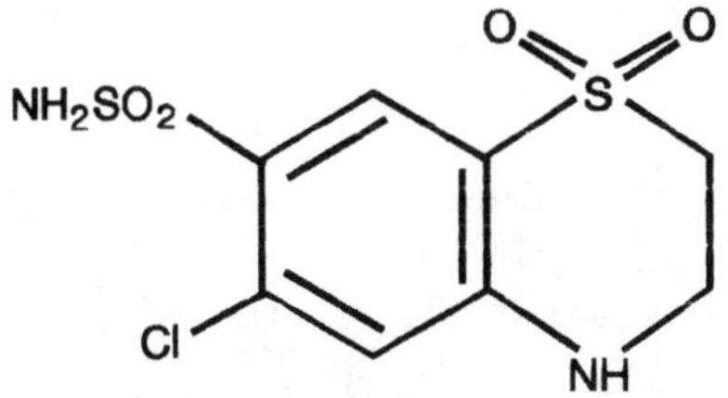

FIGURE 4-1

Chemical structure, as pictured. Chemical name: 6-chloro-3,4-dihydro-2H-1,2,4-benzothia-diazine-7-sulfonamide 1,1-dioxide. Generic name: hydrochlorothiazide (a diuretic). Trade name: Esidrix, HydroDIURIL, Oretic.

derived was first isolated near a sewer outlet in Sardinia. Streptomycin was first isolated from the stomach of a chicken. As stated in Chapter 2, many drugs still in use today were originally derived from plant sources.

2. A totally new chemical may be derived from molecular manipulation of a drug which is already in use. This new chemical may be semisynthetic or totally synthetic. With only very slight molecular changes, the original drug may be significantly changed in a variety of ways which influence absorption, metabolism, half-life, and side effects. For example, penicillin G is derived from the mold *Penicillium chrysogenum.* One of the drug's major drawbacks is that it is destroyed by stomach acid and cannot be administered orally. When the basic penicillin nucleus was changed by adding certain chemicals to the vats where the penicillin was fermenting, a semisynthetic penicillin was obtained which is not destroyed by stomach acid. This new penicillin derivative was ampicillin.

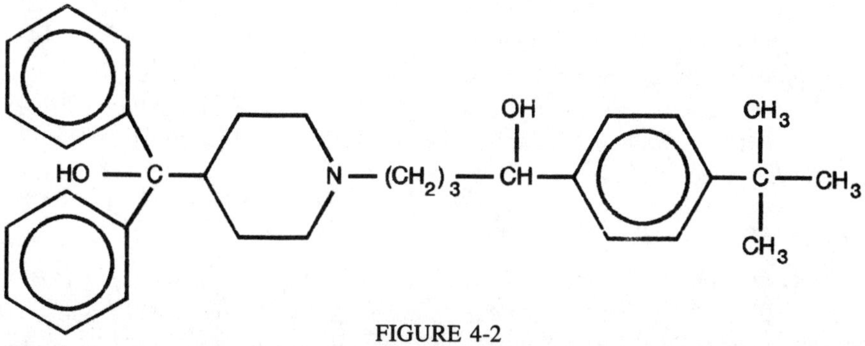

FIGURE 4-2

Chemical structure, as pictured. Chemical name: alpha-[4-(1,1-dimethylethyl)phenyl]-4-hydroxydiphenylmethyl)-1-piperidinebutanol. Generic name: terfenadine. Trade name: Seldane.

In 1957 the first benzodiazepine antianxiety drug was synthesized: chlordiazepoxide (Librium). Working with its basic molecular structure, the same researcher then produced diazepam (Valium).

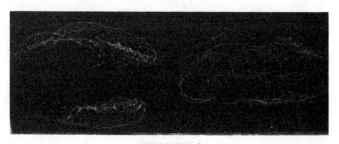

FIGURE 4-3
Computer manipulation of drugs at the molecular level.
Photo courtesy of Dana Duke, *Discover* Publications, ©1981.

Until recently, designing a new drug by changing the molecular structure of an existing drug was a slow process of trial and error, using intuition and molecular models made from wood and wire. Now, chemists use computers to aid them in designing new drugs. A computer can process hundreds of variables in chemical structure in a fraction of the time it previously took a chemist to do this manually. The computer can identify those chemicals which would probably not be successful in treating disease before time and money are invested in extensive testing. With computers, chemists can study any molecule, rotating it in three dimensions on the computer screen, as described below by Marcia Bartusiak in "Designing Drugs with Computer":

> A computer can display the molecular structure of any drug from a listing of thousands contained in its memory. By looking at and analyzing one of these stored molecules, or one built on the screen from scratch, chemists can tell if a drug's particular arrangement of atoms is the molecular "key" that fits into and opens a biological "lock" [a receptor on the cell membrane]. . . . When a chemist wants to know why different looking drugs act on the same receptor, he can ask the computer to superimpose them all on the screen so he can see how their atoms match up.
>
> *Discover* (August 1981), pp. 48-49

Recombinant DNA technology (also known as **gene splicing** or **genetic engineering**) is a new field in drug development. Aided by computer design and advances in technology, researchers are able, with the use of enzymes, to remove DNA chemically from one organism and transplant it into another organism. The recipient organism, usually a common bacterium which multiplies rapidly,* is then directed by the new DNA to produce a particular substance. In huge vats, these bacteria can produce unlimited quantities of pharmaceuticals. In 1982, human insulin (Humulin) became the first recombinant DNA drug to be approved by the FDA.

Drug Testing, Manufacturing, and Marketing

Chemical analysis of a drug done in a laboratory in test tubes is known as **in vitro testing** (Latin for *in glass*). Testing carried out in animals or humans is termed **in vivo testing** (Latin for *in the living*). No matter how a drug was originally discovered or designed, it must be thoroughly tested by the pharmaceutical manufacturer according to certain guidelines specified by the FDA to determine its effectiveness and safety.

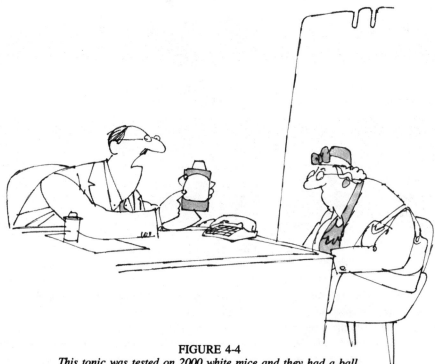

FIGURE 4-4
This tonic was tested on 2000 white mice and they had a ball.
—David W. Harbaugh
Reprinted with permission

---

*"A single bacterium can become two, then four, then eight, then a billion in less than a day. All that's needed is enough food—a standard microbiological medium—for the whole multiplying clan to eat. . . . [They then] mass-produce perfect copies of themselves, . . . continually pumping out the desired product without error." Doug Stewart, "These Germs Work Wonders," *Reader's Digest* (January 1991), pp. 83-86.

An animal phase of drug testing precedes that of human testing. During that time, any toxic effects, side effects, addiction, cancerous tumors, or fetal deformities are noted and evaluated. Also during this phase, the therapeutic index of the drug is calculated. The **therapeutic index (TI)** reflects the margin of safety between the dosage which produces a **therapeutic effect** and the dosage which produces a **toxic effect.** Animal studies, however, are not always a reliable indicator of how well a drug will perform in humans. For example, penicillin causes few side effects in humans, even in fairly high doses, but it is toxic in rather small doses in some animals. Therefore, some manufacturers are seeking alternative methods to animal testing.

EARN $400

Healthy male/female volunteers age 18 to 35 needed now to participate in upcoming inpatient studies. Stay in our pleasant dormitory at Utopia University, with recreational facilities available.

CENTER FOR VACCINE DEVELOPMENT
Utopia University

FIGURE 4-5
Typical newspaper ad for volunteers

When animal studies are completed, the pharmaceutical company applies to the FDA for permission to test the drug in humans.

There are three phases of human testing. During phase one, healthy volunteers are used to study a safe dose range, evaluate side effects, and establish a correct dosage. Absorption, metabolism, and excretion of the drug are also studied. It is not uncommon to see want ads in the classified sections of newspapers of large cities for volunteers for these drug studies. Informed consent is mandatory and, during the testing, volunteers are monitored and given medical examinations.

In phase two, the drug is given on an experimental basis to patients with the disease it will eventually be used to treat. This is done to determine the extent of its **therapeutic effect.** During phase three, the drug is administered to several hundred or several thousand ill patients in exactly the way in which it will be used clinically (dosage, route of administration) and marketed. The performance of the drug is compared to that of other drugs currently being used to treat the same disease to evaluate its effectiveness. In addition, double blind studies with the drug and a placebo are performed.

Once phase three is completed, the pharmaceutical company then submits all of its documentation on the safety and effectiveness of the drug to the FDA to await final approval for marketing. This documentation can be quite extensive. "The widely used ulcer drug cimetidine (Tagamet) is a case in point. After testing for four years, the SmithKline company had accumulated a stack of documents 17 feet high that had to be carted to the FDA in a truck," according to Denise Grady in "Bottleneck at the FDA," *Discover* (November 1981), p. 56.

It is then the responsibility of the FDA to evaluate the new drug based on the manufacturer's documentation. This process can take a year or more before final approval or rejection is given. The FDA must weigh the inherent risks of the drug against its potential benefits. For example, a drug for arthritis which produced serious side effects would not be considered desirable. However, a new chemotherapy drug, effective in treating a type of cancer which did not respond to other drugs on the market, would be desirable in spite of serious side effects.

Once a drug has received its final approval from the FDA, its ingredients, manufacturing process, labeling, packaging, and dosage cannot be changed. With further clinical trials, however, a drug's indicated uses may be expanded. For example, propranolol (Inderal) was approved by the FDA in 1967 for arrhythmias. In 1973 it was approved for treating hypertension. In 1979 it was approved to treat patients with migraine headaches.

Another example of expanded uses: The drug indomethacin (Indocin), a little-used agent for arthritis and gout, was approved in 1985 for use in premature infants to close a patent ductus arteriosus (a heart defect) to avoid surgery. Although this new clinical indication seems far removed from the drug's previous use, it is actually based on the same pharmacologic action—inhibiting the production of prostaglandins.

All pharmaceutical companies are protected by a 17-year **patent** on new drugs. This means that, during that time, no other company can manufacture or market an identical drug. However, part of the 17-year patent period is lost during the testing process before the drug is even approved by the FDA. At the end of the 17 years when the patent expires, any pharmaceutical company can manufacture that drug under its original generic name or under a new brand name which they select. The original brand name can be used only by the original manufacturer. If a generic drug is manufactured by several different pharmaceutical companies, it may be listed under different names: one generic and several trade names. For example:

Generic name: ampicillin.

Trade name: Omnipen (Wyeth-Ayerst)
Polycillin (Bristol)
Totacillin (Beecham Labs)
Amcill (Parke-Davis)
Principen (Squibb)

Because the 17-year patent protects the original manufacturer for only a brief time, manufacturers hope that their new drug will be successful and that the trade name selected will become firmly entrenched in the minds of prescribing physicians before other trade names for that generic drug can be marketed when the patent expires.

The FDA carefully monitors the quality of both generic and trade name drugs manufactured by all pharmaceutical companies. A generic drug and its related trade name drugs must contain exactly the same active drug ingredients and must be able to be administered in exactly the same way. However, the **inert ingredients** (binders, fillers) in each dose, as well as preservatives, antioxidants, and buffers used vary among manufacturers. In most cases, the effects on the disintegration and absorption of a drug are minimal; however, in some cases, the choice of ingredients does seem to affect the therapeutic action of the drug.

If the bioavailability of the active drug ingredient varies, this can be particularly crucial in drugs with a low **therapeutic index** (a low margin of safety between the therapeutic and the toxic dose). A 1971 study in the *New England Journal of Medicine* compared four preparations of digoxin. All met government standards, but the **bioavailability** of the active drug was much higher for one preparation than for the others. This resulted in blood levels of the drug which ranged from subtherapeutic with one product to toxic with another product.

Pharmacists are permitted to substitute the generic drug for a prescribed trade name drug, unless the prescribing physician specifically requests no substitutions. The use of generic rather than trade name drugs can result in considerable savings to consumers, but for certain critical drugs—such as digoxin (Lanoxin) used for congestive heart failure, and phenytoin (Dilantin) used to prevent seizures—many physicians prefer to rely on the proven therapeutic action of the trade name drug for the reasons discussed above.

REVIEW QUESTIONS

1. What are the three names that a drug can be assigned?
2. The spelling of generic drugs may be similar if they belong to the same drug classification. True or False?
3. List six ways in which pharmaceutical companies select a trade name for a drug.
4. In what two fundamental ways may a new drug be discovered?
5. In general, describe recombinant DNA technology and how it helps pharmaceutical manufacturers produce certain drugs.
6. What is meant by tests which are performed in vitro? In vivo?
7. What type of drug characteristics/effects are studied during the three phases of human testing of a drug prior to FDA approval?
8. Explain the reasoning behind some physicians' decisions not to prescribe less costly generic equivalents of certain drugs for their patients.

5

Drug Forms and
Routes of Administration

Before a drug can receive final approval by the FDA, the pharmaceutical company must clearly state in what form or forms the drug will be manufactured and what routes of administration are determined safe and effective. Different forms of a drug are appropriate for different routes of administration. Some drugs are ineffective when administered in a certain form or by a certain route; other drugs may seriously injure the patient if administered in certain forms or by a certain route.

Drug Forms

1. **Tablet.** This drug form contains dried powdered active drug as well as binders and fillers to provide bulk and ensure proper tablet size. A **scored** tablet has an indented line running across the top. It can be easily broken into two pieces with a knife to produce two doses. **Enteric** tablets are covered with a special coating which resists stomach acid but dissolves in the alkaline environment of the small intestine to avoid irritating the stomach (example: Ecotrin). **Slow-release** tablets are manufactured to provide a continuous, sustained release of certain drugs. Often this is abbreviated as SR (slow release) or LA (long acting) in the trade name of the drug (examples: Procan SR and Entex LA). **Caplets** are easy-to-swallow coated tablets in the form of capsules. Tablets can also be designed to be dissolved in water before being taken orally (example: Klorvess effervescent tablets). Some over-the-counter drugs come in the form of **lozenges.** These tablets are formed of a hardened base of sugar and water containing the drug and other flavorings. They are never swallowed, but are allowed to dissolve slowly in the mouth and release the drug topically to the tissues of the mouth and throat (example: Cepacol lozenges). In prescriptions, *tablet* is sometimes abbreviated as *tab* or *tabs.*

2. **Capsule.** This drug form comes in two varieties. The first is a soft gelatin shell manufactured in one piece in which the drug is in a liquid form inside the shell (examples: Atromid-S and fat-soluble vitamins such as A and E). The second form of capsule is a hard shell manufactured in two pieces which fit together and hold the drug which is in a powdered or granular form. Many nonprescription cold remedies and pain medications were manufactured in this form until some Tylenol capsules were reported to be contaminated with cyanide in the early 1980s. Subse-

quently, many companies now manufacture their nonprescription pain medications in a tablet or caplet form. Many prescription drugs, however, are still manufactured as capsules. In prescriptions, *capsule* is sometimes abbreviated as *cap* or *caps*.

3. **Cream.** A cream is a semisolid emulsion of oil (such as lanolin or petroleum) and water, the main ingredient being water. Emulsifying agents are added to keep the oil and water well mixed. Many topical drugs are manufactured in a cream base (example: hydrocortisone cream).

4. **Ointment.** An ointment is a semisolid emulsion of an oil (such as lanolin or petroleum) and water, the main ingredient being oil. Many topical drugs are manufactured in an ointment base (example: Kenalog ointment). Specially formulated ophthalmic ointments are made to be applied topically to the eye without causing irritation. Most creams and ointments are applied to the skin without precise measurement; however, nitroglycerin ointment (used to prevent angina) is precisely measured in inches on a specially marked applicator paper which is taped to the patient's skin.

5. **Lotion.** A lotion is a suspension of an active drug in a water base for external use (examples: Keri lotion, calamine lotion).

6. **Powder.** A powder is a finely ground form of an active drug. Powdered drugs can be contained in capsules but can also be found in glass vials where they must be reconstituted with water before being injected (example: intravenous ampicillin). Powders can also be reconstituted for oral use (example: Metamucil).

7. **Liquid.** Liquids come in the form of either solutions or suspensions. Solutions contain the drug fully dissolved in a base. Solutions never need to be mixed as the drug-to-water concentration is always the same in every part of the solution, even after prolonged standing. **Solutions** come in many forms: elixirs, syrups, tinctures, liquid sprays, and foams.

Elixirs contain an alcohol and water base with added sugar and flavoring (example: Tylenol elixir). Elixirs are commonly used for pediatric or elderly patients who cannot swallow the tablet or capsule form of a drug. **Syrups** contain no alcohol, being a concentrated solution of sugar, water, and flavorings. Syrups are sweeter and more viscous (thicker) than elixirs. Most over-the-counter cough medications have a syrup base which not only carries the drug but acts to soothe inflamed mucous membranes in the throat. **Tinctures** have an alcohol and water base (example: Merthiolate tincture).

Liquid sprays contain a solution of the drug combined with water or alcohol to be sprayed by a pump or aerosol propellant. Spray liquid drugs are commonly used for topical application (examples: Afrin nasal spray, Primatene Mist spray, Benadryl spray.) Nitroglycerin is available in a spray form for application under the tongue during anginal attacks. Certain over-the-counter contraceptives are available as **foams**.

Suspensions contain fine, undissolved particles of a drug suspended in a liquid base. After prolonged standing, these fine particles will gradually settle to the bottom of the container. Therefore it is always important to shake suspensions well before using, a fact that is noted on the label of these drugs (example: Maalox and

ᐧother antacids). An **emulsion** is a suspension in which fat particles are mixed with water (example: Intralipid intravenous fat solution).

Two general terms used to describe a liquid are **aqueous** (from the Latin word *aqua,* water), meaning of watery consistency, and **viscous,** which designates a non-watery or thick liquid.

8. Suppositories. Suppositories contain a solid base of glycerin or cocoa butter containing the drug. They are manufactured in appropriate sizes for rectal or vaginal insertion and also come in adult and pediatric sizes. Vaginal suppositories are most often used to treat vaginal infections but can also be used orally to treat yeast infections in the mouth. Rectal suppositories can be used to administer drugs to patients who are vomiting (example: Tylenol suppositories).

9. Transdermal. The transdermal form of drugs is relatively new. It consists of a multi-layered disk containing a drug reservoir, a porous membrane, and an adhesive layer to hold it to the skin. The porous membrane regulates the amount of drug released to the skin (example: Transderm-Nitro for prevention of angina). These drugs are often known as transdermal patches.

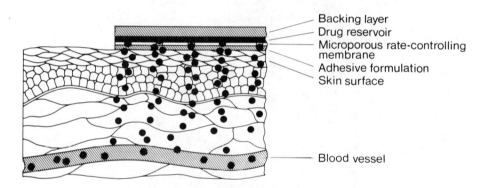

FIGURE 5-1

Cross section of a transdermal patch of Transderm-Nitro. Illustration courtesy of CIBA Pharmaceutical Company.

Routes of Administration

There are various routes of drug administration. Some drugs are approved for use via more than one route and are manufactured in different forms appropriate for those different routes. Each route of administration has distinct advantages and disadvantages as discussed below. A drug given by one route will be therapeutic; given by another route, it may be ineffective, harmful, or even fatal.

1. Oral. The oral route is the most convenient route of administration and the most commonly used. Tablets, capsules, and liquids are all given orally. Even patients who have difficulty swallowing a tablet or capsule can usually take the liquid form of a drug without problems. Infants are given drugs in a liquid form mixed with a small amount of formula in a nipple. Even unconscious patients can be given liquid medication through a nasogastric (NG) tube. The oral route is routinely abbreviated as PO or p.o. (Latin for *per os,* meaning *through the mouth).*

Disadvantages of the oral route include the following: Some drugs, most particularly certain penicillins, are inactivated by stomach acid and cannot be given orally. After oral administration, some drugs are so quickly metabolized by the liver as they pass through the portal circulation that a therapeutic blood level cannot be achieved in the systemic circulation. Therefore, these drugs can be given intravenously (example: lidocaine [Xylocaine] for cardiac arrhythmias). Some drugs cannot be taken with certain foods and drinks as they either combine chemically to form an insoluble complex or interact to produce adverse side effects (example: tetracycline cannot be taken with dairy products).

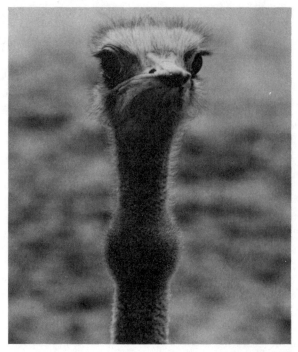

FIGURE 5-2
Some patients have difficulty swallowing solid medication. Photo courtesy of the Pharmaceutical Products Division of Abbott Laboratories, Chicago, Illinois.

2. **Sublingual.** Sublingual administration involves placing the drug (usually in a tablet form) under the tongue and allowing it to slowly dissolve. The tablet is not swallowed (this would then become oral administration). The drug is absorbed quickly through oral mucous membranes and into the large blood vessels under the tongue.

The sublingual route provides a faster therapeutic effect than the oral route (example: nitroglycerin tablets or spray for treating angina attacks).

3. **Rectal.** Absorption of a drug via the rectal route of administration is slow and often unpredictable. This route is reserved for certain clinical situations, such as when the patient is vomiting and unable to take medications which cannot be given by injection (example: Tylenol suppositories). The exception to this is when drugs are administered rectally to relieve constipation or treat hemorrhoids.

4. **Vaginal.** The vaginal route is used to treat vaginal infections and vaginitis by using creams and suppositories (examples: Monistat suppositories, Premarin vaginal cream). Over-the-counter contraceptive foams are inserted vaginally as well.

5. **Topical.** When a drug is applied directly to the skin or to the mucous membranes of the eye, ear, nose, or mouth, it is administered via the topical route. The effects of the drug are generally local, not systemic (throughout the body) (examples: bacitracin antibiotic ointment, Sudafed nasal decongestant spray, Timoptic eye drops for glaucoma).

Sites of topical administration are abbreviated as follows:

Abbreviation	Latin Meaning	Medical Meaning
A.D.	*auris dextra*	right ear
A.S.	*auris sinistra*	left ear
A.U.	*auris utraque*	both ears
O.D.	*oculus dexter*	right eye
O.S.	*oculus sinister*	left eye
O.U.	*oculus uterque*	both eyes

6. **Transdermal.** This relatively new route of administration differs from the topical route in that the drug is applied to the skin via physical delivery through a porous membrane, with the therapeutic effects felt systemically, not just at the site of administration. Drugs delivered by the transdermal route are usually manufactured in the form of a patch. (For the physical construction of a transdermal patch, refer to Figure 5-1.) Worn on the skin, the patch releases the drug slowly over a 24-hour period, providing sustained therapeutic blood levels (example: Transderm-Nitro for prevention of angina).

7. **Inhalation.** This route of administration involves the inhaling of a drug in a gas or liquid form. The drug is absorbed through the alveoli of the lungs (examples: nitrous oxide, a general anesthetic; albuterol [Proventil], a bronchodilator).

8. **Parenteral.** Parenteral is a general term, taken from the Greek words *para* and *enteron,* which literally mean *apart from the intestine.* Technically, *parenteral* means all routes of administration other than by mouth; but in clinical usage, parenteral commonly includes just the following routes of administration: intradermal, subcutaneous, intramuscular, intravenous, and the other less frequently used routes of intra-arterial and intrathecal.

Intradermal administration involves the injection of a liquid into the dermis, the layer of skin just below the epidermis. The epidermis itself is less than 1/20 of an inch thick; therefore, when an intradermal injection is correctly positioned, the tip of the needle is still plainly visible through the skin (example: Mantoux test for tuberculosis).

Subcutaneous administration involves the injection of liquid into the subcutaneous tissues, the fatty layer of tissue just under the dermis of the skin but above the muscle layer (example: insulin, heparin, allergy shots). There are few blood vessels in this layer, so drugs are absorbed more slowly than when given by intramuscular injection. Diabetics who inject insulin utilize approximately 10-12 different areas on the upper arm, thigh, and abdomen to rotate the site of daily subcutaneous insulin injections. The term *subcutaneous* is abbreviated in various ways as *subQ, SQ,* and *subcu*; there is no one official abbreviation.

Intramuscular (abbreviated *I.M.* or *IM*) administration involves the injection of a liquid into the **belly** (area of greatest mass) of a large muscle. The large muscles of the body are well supplied with blood vessels, and drugs are absorbed more quickly than following subcutaneous injection. There are only five intramuscular injection sites which can be used; other sites invite damage to adjacent nerves and blood vessels.
- Deltoid, located on the upper arm, lateral aspect.
- Vastus lateralis, located on the midthigh, lateral aspect.
- Rectus femoris, located on the midthigh, anterior aspect.
- Ventrogluteal, located on the side of the hip over the gluteus muscle.
  between the anterior superior and posterior superior spines of the iliac crest.
- Dorsogluteal, located over the gluteus minimus and edge of the gluteus
  maximus muscles in the upper outer quadrant of each buttock.

Some drugs cannot be given by intramuscular injection because they are not water soluble and will precipitate out in the intramuscular tissue (example: Valium, Librium).

Examples of drugs given intramuscularly: Demerol for pain; vitamin B_{12} for pernicious anemia; Garamycin for bacterial infections.

Intravenous (abbreviated *I.V.* or *IV*) administration of a drug involves the injection of a liquid directly into a vein and may be done in one of three ways. The injection of a single dose of a drug (**bolus**) may be given through a **port** (rubber stopper) into an existing intravenous (I.V.) line. This is often referred to as **I.V. push** because the drug is manually pushed into the I.V. line in a very short period of time. A drug may also be mixed with the fluid in an I.V. bag or bottle and administered continuously over several hours. This is known as **I.V. drip.** A drug may also be mixed in a very small I.V. bag or bottle and administered over an hour or less by I.V. drip. This small secondary I.V. bag or bottle is connected through tubing to a port in the existing primary I.V. line. This method is known as **I.V. piggyback** administration.

The therapeutic effect of many drugs given intravenously can be seen immediately. This is because the drug does not need to be absorbed from tissue or muscle into the bloodstream before it can exert an effect.

Examples of drugs given intravenously: Pentothal for induction of general anesthesia; Valium for control of continuous epileptic seizures; chemotherapy drugs; antibiotics.

Other parenteral routes which have specialized uses include:

Intra-articular. This route is used only to inject specific drugs, such as corticosteroids, into the joint to decrease inflammation and pain.

Intracardiac. This route is used only during emergency resuscitation measures (example: Adrenalin is given to directly stimulate the heart muscle during cardiac arrest).

Endotracheal. This route is used only during emergency resuscitation measures (example: Adrenalin).

Intrathecal. *Theca* (actually *theka*) is Greek for *sheath.* Intrathecal administration involves the injection of a liquid within the sheath or meninges of the spinal cord into the cerebrospinal fluid (example: spinal anesthesia).

Intra-arterial. This route is used occasionally for direct injection of a chemotherapeutic agent to a tumor area. Generally, arterial lines are used for continuous monitoring of blood pressure and are not used to administer drugs.

Umbilical artery or vein catheter. This route is accessible only in newborn infants and is used to administer fluids and draw blood. It is generally not used to give drugs. Instead, an I.V. line inserted peripherally (in the hand, foot, or scalp) is used for drug administration.

REVIEW QUESTIONS

1. What is the reason for manufacturing a drug as an enterically coated tablet?
2. What are caplets?
3. Besides tablets and capsules, list five other forms in which drugs are manufactured.
4. Describe the difference between an elixir, a syrup, and a tincture base for drugs.
5. List two disadvantages encountered when administering some drugs by the oral route.
6. The sublingual route of administration provides more rapid absorption of a drug than the oral route. True or False?
7. Give the meaning of the abbreviations A.S. and O.U.
8. A diabetic would inject insulin via what route of administration?
9. Describe three of the five acceptable sites for an intramuscular injection.
10. Differentiate between the I.V. push, I.V. drip, and I.V. piggyback methods of administration.

SPELLING TIPS

- lozenge (no final r, although it is commonly mispronounced "lozenger").
- intravenous (not intervenous). Note same with intra-articular, intra-arterial, intracardiac, intradermal, intramuscular, and intrathecal. *Intra* means *within. Inter* means *between.*

6

Steps in the Drug Cycle

Following administration, most drugs go through several steps in a well-defined sequence before being excreted from the body. These steps include:

Absorption from the site of administration
Distribution via the circulatory system
Metabolism
Excretion from the body

Absorption

Absorption involves the movement of the drug from the site of administration through tissues into the bloodstream. Topical drugs, however, are not absorbed to any great extent, and their therapeutic action is exerted locally at the site of administration. For other drugs, absorption involves several steps.

Tablets or capsules first disintegrate; this step is omitted with drugs in the liquid form. Then the drug is dissolved in body fluids (saliva, gastric juice, or tissue fluid) and absorbed into blood vessels. The presence or absence of food in the stomach can influence the rate of absorption.

Some drugs are not absorbed at all following oral administration (example: the antibiotics neomycin and kanamycin). This drawback can be overcome by administering these drugs via a different route.

This same property of nonabsorption via the oral route can be used to an advantage with other drugs. For example, Carafate is given orally to bind directly to stomach ulcers. It is not absorbed. Neomycin may be given orally to exert its antibiotic effect solely in the intestinal tract prior to abdominal surgery. Metamucil is not absorbed but binds with water in the intestinal tract to increase stool bulk and relieve constipation.

Following administration of a drug by inhalation, the vaporized liquid is absorbed through the mucous membrane lining the alveoli and into adjacent capillaries. Some drugs given by inhalation exert a topical effect but also may have systemic side effects (example: Alupent bronchodilator). Inhaled general anesthetic gases exert only a systemic effect.

Following rectal or vaginal administration, a suppository or cream melts and releases the drug topically to the mucous membranes. The rate of absorption with rectal administration is rather slow and variable; therefore, it is reserved for topical

28

drug applications (to treat hemorrhoids, for example) unless other routes of administration are unavailable (such as when a patient is vomiting and the drug is not manufactured in a form which can be given I.M. or I.V.).

Injections (intradermal, subcutaneous, intramuscular) of liquid drugs are absorbed from body tissues into adjacent capillaries. Only intravenous injections entirely bypass the step of absorption because the drug is administered directly into the bloodstream.

Distribution

Once a drug has been absorbed into the bloodstream, it is distributed throughout the body via the circulatory system. As a drug dose enters the bloodstream, some of the drug binds to circulating **plasma proteins** (such as **albumin**). Plasma proteins have indentations in their molecular surfaces which permit drug molecules to bind to them. Drug molecules bound to plasma proteins are essentially pharmacologically inactive. As the portion of the drug which did not bind to plasma proteins moves from the blood into body tissues, some of the bound drug is released from the plasma proteins to maintain an equilibrium.

The portion of unbound drug which moves into body tissues comes in contact with cell membranes where it exerts an effect by interacting with a receptor. This process will be discussed in the next chapter.

One area of the body where many drugs may not be distributed following absorption is in the central nervous system. The brain tissues are protected to some extent by the so-called **blood-brain barrier** which theoretically exists between the capillary wall of blood vessels in the brain and surrounding brain tissues. Some drugs, such as antihistamines, and morphine-type drugs, are able to pass through the blood-brain barrier and cause effects such as drowsiness and euphoria, respectively. General anesthetics also cross the blood-brain barrier to produce unconsciousness.

Sometimes the blood-brain barrier actually excludes the very drugs needed to correct disease conditions in the brain. Parkinson disease is due to a deficiency of the **neurotransmitter dopamine** in certain areas of the brain. While dopamine can be administered orally, it cannot cross the blood-brain barrier to be therapeutically effective. Fortunately, another drug, levodopa, is structurally different and can cross the blood-brain barrier where it is then converted to dopamine to correct the deficiency.

At one time it was thought that the placenta formed a barrier to protect the developing fetus from harmful drugs. It is now known that the placenta allows nearly all drugs to pass from the maternal circulation through to the fetus. Each year, many infants are born addicted or with birth defects due to the action of drugs.

Metabolism

Metabolism is also known as **biotransformation** because, in this process, a drug circulating in the bloodstream is transformed or metabolized from its original active form to a less active or even inactive form. This process is accomplished by the action of enzymes.

A few drugs, such as chloral hydrate (Noctec), a sedative, are actually administered in an inactive form and remain so until they are metabolized. It is the **metabolite** of this drug which actually possesses pharmacologic activity.

The liver is the principal organ of metabolism, although other organs metabolize certain drugs to a limited degree. Drugs absorbed through the mucous membrane of the stomach or intestines enter the bloodstream via the portal vein. Before this vein empties into the general circulation, it passes through the liver. Therefore, drugs given by the oral route and absorbed from the GI tract are immediately exposed to metabolism by liver enzymes. The metabolic action of the liver is referred to as the **first-pass effect**—the drug first passes through the liver before reaching the general circulation to exert any systemic effect. For some drugs, the first-pass effect is so extensive that almost all of the drug dose is immediately metabolized. These drugs are not given by oral administration because no therapeutic effect can be achieved (example: lidocaine [Xylocaine]). Some drugs are never metabolized at all and are excreted unchanged through the kidneys (example: Garamycin).

Because the liver is the principal organ of metabolism for most drugs, a decreased rate of drug metabolism can occur in those patients with liver diseases and hepatitis. Drug dosages for these patients need to be adjusted downward in order to compensate for the prolonged pharmacologic action of unmetabolized drug in the bloodstream. In elderly patients, the dosages of certain drugs need to be reduced because of impaired liver function brought on by the degenerative changes associated with aging. Premature infants have very immature livers which are unable to metabolize drugs efficiently. The dosage of their drugs must be carefully calculated to avoid toxicity.

Excretion

The excretion of drugs is a necessary step in ridding the body of waste products (inactive drug **metabolites**) or removing active drugs which are not metabolized by the liver. The principal organ involved in the excretion of drugs is the kidney, although other organs are involved to a limited degree. The lungs excrete certain general anesthetics as the patient exhales. Also trace amounts of drugs are excreted in saliva, tears, and most importantly, breast milk. While the amount of drug excreted in breast milk may be insignificant when compared to the total amount of drug excreted by the kidneys, it can cause significant effects in the nursing baby if the drug remains in its active form.

A drug is not automatically excreted by the kidney when it reaches that point in the circulatory system. Some portion of the drug still remains bound to plasma proteins such as albumin. Albumin is a large molecule which does not readily filter through the normal glomerulus. Therefore, that portion of the drug bound to albumin passes through the glomerulus and is returned to the general circulation. However, unbound portions of the drug are small enough to be filtered through the glomerulus.

But even when a drug has reached the nephron of the kidney, it still may not be automatically excreted in the urine. At this point a further distinction is made between **water-soluble drugs** and **fat-soluble drugs.** Water-soluble drugs are filtered through the nephron and immediately excreted in the urine because of their affinity for water. Fat-soluble (lipid) drugs are not readily excreted in the urine because they are more attracted to the lipid structure of the renal tubule wall than to the water base of urine. Lipid-soluble drugs are returned to the general circulation where they eventually undergo metabolism by the liver into a more water-soluble form which is then excreted. Without the action of the liver, it would be difficult for a lipid-soluble drug to ever be excreted by the kidneys. Indeed, it has been estimated that some barbiturates which are lipid soluble would remain in the bloodstream for years if the liver did not metabolize them to a water-soluble form.

Poor renal function can significantly prolong the effects of some drugs. Patients with renal disease and elderly patients with physiologically decreased levels of kidney function are prescribed lower dosages of drugs to prevent toxic symptoms due to decreased rates of drug excretion.

REVIEW QUESTIONS

1. Describe the route of absorption, distribution, metabolism, and excretion of a drug administered orally.
2. What is meant by the first-pass effect?
3. How do plasma proteins such as albumin regulate the amount of drug circulating in the bloodstream?
4. What is the proposed function of the blood-brain barrier?
5. Why are drug dosages decreased for elderly patients?
6. Give two reasons why drugs reaching the kidney may not be excreted immediately in the urine.

7

Drug Effects

Drugs exert their effects in a number of ways and at a number of sites within the body. In this chapter, we will explore:

> Local versus systemic effects
> Therapeutic effects
> Side effects
> Toxic effects
> Allergic effects
> Receptors: sites of effects
> Drug interactions

Local Versus Systemic Effects

Basically, drugs act in one of two ways, either locally or systemically to exert both therapeutic and side effects. A local effect is limited to the site of administration and those tissues immediately surrounding it. Drugs applied topically generally exert a local effect (example: nasal sprays, topical creams and ointments).

A systemic effect is not limited to the site of administration but can be felt throughout the body to varying degrees. Drugs taken intravenously and intramuscularly always exert a systemic effect. Drugs taken orally and subcutaneously usually exert a systemic effect. Inhaled drugs may exert either mainly a local effect or a systemic one depending on the drug and its dosage. Drugs given vaginally exert a local effect. Drugs given rectally may exert either a local or a systemic effect, depending on the drug.

The same drug given via different routes can exert either a local or a systemic effect. For example, lidocaine (Xylocaine) in a viscous solution is gargled for topical anesthesia, injected subcutaneously for local anesthesia, or given intravenously to act systemically in treating cardiac arrhythmias. The antihistamine diphenhydramine (Benadryl) can be purchased over the counter orally and as a spray or cream for topical application to relieve itching; it can also be prescribed orally in a capsule to act systemically to relieve allergic symptoms.

However, many medical problems and diseases cannot be treated by drugs which act only locally at the site of administration. Treatment of major illnesses such as cardiac disease, mental illness, and diabetes must be done with drugs which act systemically. In acting systemically these drugs exert an effect on the **target organ** (the heart, for example, in congestive heart failure); however, they also exert effects on other organs as well. The effect exerted on the target organ is termed the therapeutic effect. The effects exerted on other organs can be divided into several types of effects, as discussed below.

Therapeutic and Side Effects

The therapeutic effect is the drug's main action for which it was prescribed by the physician. The therapeutic effect of the drug is selected to cure a disease (example: antibiotics), decrease disease symptoms (example: insulin), or prevent a disease (example: vaccines). The perfect drug would have a complete therapeutic effect perfectly suited to its medical purpose, with no side effects. Unfortunately, the perfect drug does not exist.

The therapeutic effect is not always exerted on a **target organ,** as described above. With antibiotics, the therapeutic effect involves the destruction or inhibition of pathogenic (disease-causing) bacteria within the body.

A drug is prescribed for its therapeutic effects, but if it acts systemically, it will exert effects not only on the target organ but also on other body tissues. Drug effects other than the therapeutic effect are termed side effects. Side effects can be mild and short-lived, moderate and annoying, or severe enough that the drug must be discontinued.

A list of common side effects is developed as a new drug is tested before marketing. If the side effects are severe, the FDA may not approve the drug. Once on the market, the advertisements and other informational literature connected with the drug must list these side effects.

Examples of side effects vary widely with the type of drug administered. Common gastrointestinal side effects include anorexia, nausea, vomiting, or diarrhea. Common central nervous system side effects include drowsiness, excitement, or depression. Some drugs produce few side effects, but most are associated with at least one or two side effects which are frequently observed after administration of the drug. Aspirin is well known for causing stomach irritation. A common side effect of codeine is constipation. Some antidepressant medications cause significant side effects of blurred vision, dry mouth, and fatigue. Common side effects of chemotherapy drugs may include nausea, vomiting, chills, fever, and loss of hair.

Sometimes one of the side effects of a drug can become the therapeutic effect. Many antihistamines, when given orally for allergies, produce significant drowsiness. This side effect is undesirable, particularly with patients who must drive or operate machinery. However, this side effect of drowsiness can be utilized as a therapeutic effect when an antihistamine is incorporated into a medication for insomnia. Antihistamines are a common ingredient in over-the-counter sleep aids.

Severe side effects are often referred to as **adverse effects.** Physicians may report adverse effects, some of which only become apparent after a drug is marketed and consumed by large numbers of patients, using a special form provided by the FDA. In 1986, the FDA received reports of over 53,000 adverse drug reactions. Nearly 25% of these resulted in hospitalization or death. Adverse reactions are "the seventh leading cause of hospitalization among elderly, costing $4.5 billion a year. In a recent study in the *Archives of Internal Medicine*, 5% of hospital admissions for a large metropolitan teaching hospital over a two-month period could be attributed primarily to adverse drug reactions." ("Implications of Adverse Drug Reactions," *CPN Nurse News,* Vol. 3, No. 1 [Summer 1987], p. 1.)

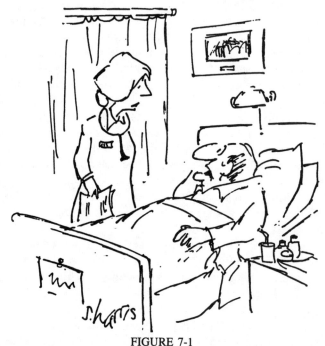

FIGURE 7-1
I stopped taking the medicine because I prefer the original disease to the side effects.
—Sidney Harris, ©1981, *American Scientist* magazine
Reprinted with permission

Toxic Effects

Toxic effects result when serum levels of a drug rise above the therapeutic level to higher levels which are toxic. Before FDA approval, the pharmaceutical manufacturer must show that a drug does not produce toxic effects when administered in therapeutic doses. However, when using a drug with a low **therapeutic index** (a narrow margin of safety between the therapeutic dose and the toxic dose) such as digoxin (Lanoxin), it is not uncommon to see toxic symptoms, particularly in elderly patients whose liver and kidneys are less able to metabolize and excrete drugs.

When toxic symptoms occur, the physician may elect to decrease the dosage of a drug, lengthen the time between doses, or discontinue the drug altogether. Patients on drugs which are known to frequently cause toxic effects are also often scheduled for blood tests to monitor drug levels and other laboratory tests to monitor particular organs which are affected. The antibiotics gentamicin (Garamycin) and kanamycin (Kantrex) are known to exert toxic effects on the ear (**ototoxicity**) and kidneys (**nephrotoxicity**). Patients on these drugs are given audiograms to monitor hearing acuity; their BUN and creatinine are also monitored to assess kidney function.

Allergic Effects

Allergic reactions are also a type of side effect but differ from side effects, adverse effects, or toxic effects in that there is a different underlying cause: the systemic release of **histamine** which occurs even when a drug is at therapeutic levels. The term *allergy* was introduced in the early 1900s. It describes a reaction which occurs when the body's immune system identifies a foreign substance (an antigen) and initiates an antibody response against it with the release of histamine. The antigen (pollen, dust, or a drug) does not produce an allergic reaction in all people, but in hypersensitive people, the presence of an **antigen** combined with an **antibody** provokes the release of **histamine** which forms the basis for all allergic symptoms. Histamine produces mild to severe allergic symptoms, depending on the amount released.

Mild allergic reactions are characterized by symptoms of itching, swelling, redness, sneezing, and wheezing. Severe to life-threatening allergic reactions involve bronchospasm, edema, shock, and death. The severest symptoms of an allergic reaction are collectively termed **anaphylaxis** or **anaphylactic shock.**

Anaphylactic shock is not a common drug reaction but is often associated with the antibiotic penicillin, although other drugs may also produce it. Interestingly, a patient may take several courses of penicillin before any allergic reaction occurs. Once a patient is sensitized to a particular drug, even a small dose can trigger an allergic reaction. In addition, some drugs show cross allergies with other drug groups because of similarities in molecular structure. For example, patients allergic to penicillin avoid other drugs in the penicillin group, such as ampicillin, and may also exhibit hypersensitivity to cephalosporin antibiotics, such as Keflex, Velosef, and Ceclor, due to their similar chemical structure.

Drug Idiosyncrasy

The term *drug idiosyncrasy* describes a drug reaction which is not a common side effect and is not based on an allergic reaction. It is an individual's unique reaction to a drug and is different from common side effects identified with the drug. A drug idiosyncrasy may have its basis in genetics. Certain genetic factors may be responsible for variations in metabolism and action of a drug. This has been supported by some evidence: "It has been demonstrated that after an identical oral dose of a given tricyclic antidepressant agent, the variation in blood concentration of the pharmacologically active drug may vary as much as 10- to 40-fold in different human subjects." (Michael C. Gerald, *Pharmacology: An Introduction to Drugs,* 2nd ed. [Englewood Cliffs, N.J.: Prentice-Hall, Inc., 1981], p. 340.)

Malignant hyperthermia (uncontrolled elevated body temperature) occurs in one out of 20,000 patients given the inhaled general anesthetic halothane because of a genetically determined chemical reaction. Unless quickly treated, malignant hyperthermia can result in death.

The Basis of Drug Effects

Most drug effects are mediated through the agency of a **receptor**. A receptor is a special protein molecule on the cell membrane specifically designed to interact with natural body chemicals; it can also interact with drugs. There are many types of receptors located on specific organs and tissues throughout the body.

One may think of a receptor as a type of lock and the drug as a key. A certain drug can unlock (or activate) a receptor. In fact, several drugs may be able to unlock one type of receptor. For example, chemically similar drugs may activate the same receptor to produce similar effects. A drug which is able to unlock or activate a receptor and produce an effect is known as an **agonist.**

Some drugs appear to fit a certain receptor but cannot actually unlock or activate the receptor to produce a pharmacological effect. These drugs are known as **antagonists.** This situation is similar to inserting the wrong key into a lock. The key may fit but cannot be turned to unlock the lock. An antagonist drug may fit with a receptor but it does not activate it. Instead, its therapeutic action is to occupy the receptor site and block other drugs from entering to activate the receptor.

It should also be noted that one drug can act as a master key to unlock several different receptors in different organs. This action accounts for the various effects (therapeutic and side effects) throughout the body that can be produced by one drug .

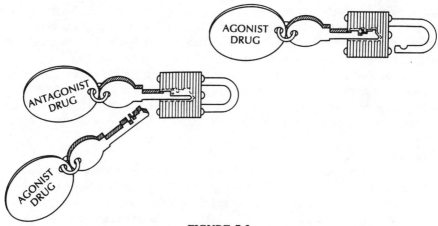

FIGURE 7-2

How agonist and antagonist drugs work. An agonist drug (key) unlocks or activates a receptor (lock). An antagonist drug (key) occupies a receptor (lock) but does not activate it.

There are many types of receptors throughout the body. **Adrenergic receptors** are part of the sympathetic nervous system and are activated by the natural **neurotransmitters epinephrine, norepinephrine,** and **dopamine** or by drugs. There are three types of adrenergic receptors (**alpha, beta$_1$,** and **beta$_2$**), which will be discussed later in this book in connection with the particular drugs which either activate or block them. **Cholinergic receptors** are part of the parasympathetic nervous system and are activated by the natural **neurotransmitter acetylcholine.** Other body chemicals (such as histamine) act on other receptors, known as **H₁ and H₂ receptors**.

Drug-Drug Interactions

Many patients are treated with more than one drug at a time. In particular, elderly patients with chronic medical problems may consume a number of medications several times a day. In addition, many patients mix prescription drugs with several over-the-counter drugs of their own choice.

When administered simultaneously, some drugs react to each other in a particular way to either accentuate or diminish the action of each. **Synergism** involves two drugs combining to produce an effect greater than the independent effects of each. Tylenol may be given with codeine to provide more complete pain relief than either can separately. A potassium-wasting diuretic may be combined with a potassium-sparing diuretic to achieve effective water loss as well as conserve potassium loss.

However, an undesirable type of synergism can occur when two drugs are given together. One well-publicized undesirable drug combination is that of alcohol and tranquilizers or alcohol and antihistamines. In both cases the drug side effect of drowsiness is heightened by the sedative effect of alcohol, often with fatal results.

Another type of drug-drug reaction is known as **antagonism.** This involves two drugs combining to produce an effect which is less than the intended effect for either drug. When the antibiotic tetracycline is taken with antacids, they combine to form an insoluble complex which prevents the tetracycline from exerting a therapeutic effect.

Antagonistic drug-food interactions also occur. Tetracycline cannot be given with milk because it also causes the formation of an insoluble complex. MAO inhibitors, a class of antidepressant drugs, cannot be given with foods rich in the amino acid tyramine because of a chemical reaction which results in hypertension, headaches, and possible stroke. These incompatible foods include aged cheeses, alcoholic beverages, bananas, liver, avocados, and chocolate.

REVIEW QUESTIONS

1. Describe the difference between local and systemic drug effects.
2. Give an example of a drug which can act either locally or systemically to produce a therapeutic effect depending on the route of administration.
3. Differentiate between a drug's therapeutic effect and its side effect.
4. List several common side effects for the GI tract and the central nervous system.
5. How does a toxic effect differ from a side effect?
6. Define the term *therapeutic index.*
7. What is the basis for all of the symptoms associated with an allergic reaction?
8. Describe the lock-and-key concept as it pertains to a drug and a receptor.
9. Give an example of a synergistic drug-drug interaction; of an antagonistic drug-drug or drug-food interaction.

8

Drug Terminology

This chapter contains detailed definitions for terminology associated with pharmacology and the administration of drugs.

acetylcholine The principal neurotransmitter of the parasympathetic nervous system, acetylcholine activates cholinergic receptor sites throughout the body. Its action is blocked by anticholinergic drugs.

addiction An acquired physical or psychological dependence on a drug with the tendency to increase its dose to provide desired effects. Drugs with addictive potential are legally referred to as controlled substances or schedule drugs.

adrenergic A type of receptor for the sympathetic nervous system, it is activated by the neurotransmitters norepinephrine, epinephrine, and dopamine. There are three common types of adrenergic receptors which are often mentioned in pharmacology: alpha adrenergic receptors, beta$_1$ (β_1) adrenergic receptors, and beta$_2$ (β_2) adrenergic receptors.

ampule A small slender glass container with a narrow neck, the ampule contains certain liquid drugs for injection or intravenous use only. The ampule is broken open by placing an alcohol swab around the neck and briskly snapping both ends of the ampule. An ampule contains enough drug for one dose. Once opened, it cannot be resealed and thus is not saved or reused. Ampules often contain drugs for emergency resuscitation, such as calcium chloride, epinephrine (Adrenalin), or 50% dextrose (D50). Ampule has no proper abbreviation and should always be written in full, although it may be dictated as *amp*. (Sample dictation: "The patient was given an amp of D50 with relief of her hypoglycemic symptoms.")

analgesic A drug that selectively suppresses pain without producing sedation.

analogue A drug which is obtained by slight molecular modification of another drug for the purpose of

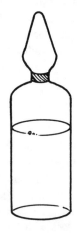

FIGURE 8-1

Ampule

38

changing certain of the original drug's characteristics to produce a new improved drug with perhaps fewer side effects or more therapeutic action. Also spelled *analog*.

anesthetic, general A drug that eliminates pain and voluntary muscle control by inducing unconsciousness.

anesthetic, local A drug that eliminates pain perception in a limited area by local action on sensory nerves.

antibiotic A drug used to treat infections by killing pathogenic bacteria.

anticholinergic Drugs which oppose the action of acetylcholine (a neurotransmitter for the parasympathetic nervous system) at the site of cholinergic receptors. Anticholinergic drugs exert a predictable set of side effects called anticholinergic effects. The ABCs of anticholinergic side effects: A—anticholinergic. B—blurred vision; bladder retention. C—constipation. D—dry mouth.

antidepressant A psychotherapeutic drug that produces mood elevation.

antiemetic A drug that prevents vomiting. (*Emesis* means *vomiting*.)

antifungal A drug used to treat fungal infections.

antihistamine A drug used to decrease the symptoms of inflammation caused by histamine released during an allergic reaction.

antihypertensive A drug that lowers high blood pressure.

anti-inflammatory A drug used to decrease the symptoms of inflammation by inhibiting the release of prostaglandins. This term is always hyphenated.

antineoplastic A drug that is selectively toxic to rapidly dividing cells such as malignant cells.

antipruritic A drug that prevents or relieves itching. (*Pruritus* means *itching*.)

antiseptic A drug which inhibits the growth of bacteria without destroying them. Antiseptics are used topically, not internally.

antispasmodic A drug used to stop the spasm of voluntary or involuntary muscles.

antitussive A drug that suppresses coughing.

antiviral A drug used to treat viral infections.

bactericidal Acting to kill bacteria. Most antibiotics are bactericidal. (Note: There is no *o* in this term, as there is in *bacteriostatic*.)

bacteriostatic Acting to inhibit the growth of bacteria but does not kill them. Bacteriostatic agents are added to drug solutions.

bioavailability That portion of the total drug dose which, after absorption, is actually available to interact with receptors and produce a therapeutic effect. Bioavailability is determined by a number of factors including drug composition (inert fillers and buffers), particle size, and stomach pH.

bore See *needle*.

bronchodilator A drug that dilates the bronchi of the lungs to increase air flow.

butterfly needle See *needle*.

cholinergic A type of receptor for the parasympathetic nervous system, it is activated by the neurotransmitter acetylcholine.

corticosteroid Topical or oral drug used to decrease inflammation.

CR An abbreviation for *controlled release*. A part of the trade name of sustained release, long-acting drugs (example: Norpace CR).

decongestant A drug that decreases congestion of the mucous membranes of the sinuses and nose.

dextrorotary A term used to describe a drug's molecules which are arranged in such a way as to bend polarized light which passes through them to the right. The word *dexter* is Latin for *right*. The generic name of some drugs indicates that they are dextrorotary: dextromethorphan, dextroamphetamine. See *isomer*.

diluent An agent such as sterile normal saline or sterile water which is used to reconstitute the powdered form of a drug to prepare it for injection. For example, **bacteriostatic diluent** has a preservative added to it to retard bacterial growth. The word *diluent* is frequently misspelled and mispronounced as *dilutent* because of its association with *dilute*.

disinfectant An agent (not used as a drug) that kills microorganisms. Used to sterilize instruments, etc.

diuretic A drug used to treat edema and hypertension by causing the kidneys to excrete more sodium and water.

drug of choice A drug which has been shown to be of particular clinical value in treating a specific disease state. It is preferred above all other similar drugs because of its superior therapeutic results. For example, digoxin (Lanoxin) is the drug of choice in treating congestive heart failure.

drug tolerance A decreased susceptibility to the effects of a drug because of continued use.

DS An abbreviation for *double-strength*. A part of the trade name of some drugs given at a double dosage in one tablet or capsule (example: Bactrim DS).

Duracap A registered trademark of Russ pharmaceutical company, it designates a time-release capsule (example: Theobid Duracap).

expectorant A drug that thins mucus in the respiratory tract to make it easier to cough up.

Extentabs A registered trademark of Robins pharmaceutical company, it designates a time-release tablet (example: Dimetapp Extentabs).

gauge See *needle*.

Gyrocaps A registered trademark of Rorer pharmaceutical company, it designates a slow-release capsule (example: Slo-Phyllin Gyrocaps).

half-life The time required for drug levels in the serum to decrease from 100% to 50%. The half-life of a drug can be significantly prolonged when liver or kidney disease results in decreased metabolism and excretion of a drug. The shorter a drug's half-life, the more frequently it must be administered to sustain therapeutic levels. Drugs with a short half-life may be manufactured in a slow-release form to provide sustained drug levels with less frequent doses. For example, procainamide has a short half-life of only two to three hours; it is manufactured in a sustained release form as Procan SR. Digoxin (Lanoxin) has a half-life of approximately 30 hours. Elderly patients with decreased liver and kidney function often develop toxicity because circulating levels of the active drug remain high for so long.

hypodermic A nonspecific term used for any injection administered below the skin.

Infatabs A registered trademark of Parke-Davis pharmaceutical company, it designates a chewable tablet with a pediatric-size dosage of a drug (example: Dilantin Infatabs).

insulin syringe A special syringe designed to measure only insulin, it is calibrated in units, not in milliliters as are all other syringes.

isomer A drug having the same molecular formula and identical atoms and numbers of atoms as another drug, but having those atoms arranged in a different way, either with different chemical bonds or in a different structural arrangement. Dextrorotary and levorotary drugs are isomers with identical chemical structures. Their major difference is their ability to reflect polarized light in opposite directions because their chemical structures are mirror images of each other. This has significance because, in one case (that of the dextro and levo isomers of amphetamine) the dextro isomer is several times more potent than the levo isomer as a central nervous system stimulant. (M. C. Gerald, *Pharmacology: An Introduction to Drugs,* 2nd ed. [Englewood Cliffs, N.J.: Prentice-Hall, Inc., 1981], p. 302.)

Kapseal A registered trademark of Parke-Davis pharmaceutical company, it designates a banded capsule.

LA An abbreviation for *long-acting.* A part of the trade name of sustained-release, long-acting drugs (example: Entex LA).

levorotary A term used to describe a drug's molecules which are arranged in a way which bends polarized light to the left. *Levo* means *left* (*laevus* is Latin for *left*). The generic name of some drugs (example: levodopa) indicates that they are levorotary. Levorotary can be abbreviated *L* as in L-dopa and L-asparaginase. See *isomer.*

loading dose If a therapeutic effect of a drug is desired immediately to treat a medical crisis, a large dose may be administered at once. The loading dose is generally twice the maintenance dose. This promptly raises the serum levels of the drug to the therapeutic range to initiate treatment. Digoxin (Lanoxin) is often given in a loading dose for patients in acute congestive heart failure. The loading dose is given only once; the maintenance dose is then used for subsequent treatment. See *maintenance dose.*

maintenance dose The maintenance dose is the standard dose prescribed by the physician for any drug. The maintenance dose is generally one-half the loading dose. See *loading dose.*

mydriatic A drug that dilates the pupil of the eye.

needle Needles are classified according to gauge and length. The **gauge** is the inside diameter of the needle. The lower the gauge number, the larger the inside diameter will be. For example, a 15-gauge needle is used for blood donation to allow the blood to flow freely through the needle to decrease turbulence and damage to the red blood cells. An 18- to 22-gauge needle is selected for intramuscular injections in adults. A 25- or 27-gauge needle is selected for starting an intravenous line on a premature infant. The inside diameter of a needle is also known as the bore. **Bore** is synonymous with *gauge* but the bore of a needle is is never assigned a number during the manufacturing process. The bore of a needle is designated as either small or large. (Sample dictation: "A large bore I.V. was inserted and normal saline allowed to run in.") A **butterfly needle** is a specially designed needle of short length and high gauge with color-coded tabs of plastic on each side of the needle. These tabs facilitate control of the needle during insertion; their appearance is like the wings of a butterfly on each side of the needle, hence the name. Butterfly needles are most often used to start intravenous lines on premature infants or on elderly patients with poor veins.

pathogen An agent (bacteria, virus, etc.) which causes disease.

peak levels Determined by a blood test, peak levels indicate the highest serum level achieved following a single dose of a drug. Peak levels are used to determine if serum levels of a drug are too high, which would result in toxic symptoms, or not high enough to produce a therapeutic effect.

placebo The term *placebo* means *I shall please* in Latin. A placebo, of itself, exerts no pharmacologic action. It exerts no therapeutic effect and produces no side effects. Placebos are used in **double-blind research studies** in which neither the researcher nor the subject knows whether the medication given to the patient was the drug being tested or a placebo. Placebos are commonly sugar pills or injections of sterile normal saline solution. Interestingly, while it is physiologically impossible for a placebo to exert any pharmacologic effect, patients often report a decrease in certain types of symptoms and can even experience "side effects" when given a placebo. These effects are quite real and demonstrate that, in some situations, the power of suggestion can produce changes within the body which closely mimic the pharmacologic action of an actual drug.

prophylaxis From a Greek word meaning *to keep guard before,* a prophylactic agent is one which is administered before the onset of disease or other condition to prevent its occurrence (example: birth control pills, flu shots, and vaccines; penicillin G is given prophylactically to patients with a history of rheumatic heart disease prior to undergoing surgery or a tooth extraction).

prototype The original type or kind of a drug from which all other drugs in that same category were developed. For example, chlorpromazine (Thorazine) is the prototype of all phenothiazine derivatives used to treat psychosis. The prototype drug does not always remain the drug of choice for treatment. It may be replaced by newer drugs.

racemic This term describes a drug which is composed of equal amounts of dextrorotary and levorotary isomers. (Sample dictation: "The patient was treated with racemic epi.") ("Epi" is a slang term for epinephrine.)

Repetabs A registered trademark of Schering pharmaceutical company, it designates a sustained-release tablet (example: Trinalin Repetabs).

SA An abbreviation for *sustained action.* A part of the trade name of sustained release, long-acting drugs (example: Choledyl SA).

Sequels A registered trademark of Lederle Laboratories, it designates a slow-release capsule (example: Ferro-Sequels).

SL An abbreviation for *sublingual.* A part of the trade name for tablets administered sublingually (example: Isordil SL).

Spansules A registered trademark of SmithKline pharmaceutical company, it designates a slow-release capsule (example: Compazine Spansules).

Sprinkle A registered trademark of Schering pharmaceutical company, it designates a long-acting capsule that can be swallowed, or the capsule can be opened and the granules of the drug can be sprinkled on food and eaten (example: Theo-Dur Sprinkle).

SR An abbreviation for *slow release* or *sustained release.* A part of the trade name of sustained release, long-acting drugs (example: Procan SR).

TB syringe See *tuberculin syringe.*

Tembids A registered trademark of Wyeth-Ayerst pharmaceutical company, it designates a sustained-release tablet (example: Isordil Tembids).

therapeutic index The therapeutic index is calculated during animal testing of any new drug. The therapeutic index reflects the relative margin of safety inherent between the dose needed to produce a therapeutic effect and the dose which produces toxic effects. The higher the therapeutic index, the better, because it indicates that the drug has a wide margin of safety. For example, penicillin has a therapeutic index of greater than 100. The therapeutic index of digoxin (Lanoxin) is less than 2, and it is not uncommon for patients being given a therapeutic dose of digoxin to begin to exhibit symptoms of toxicity.

Titradose A registered trademark of Wyeth-Ayerst pharmaceutical company, it designates a scored tablet which can be divided into smaller doses, allowing the physician to **titrate** the dose.

titrate Determining the smallest dosage that will produce the desired therapeutic effect for one particular individual.

trough levels Determined by a blood test, trough levels indicate the lowest serum level of a drug which occurs just before the next dose is to be given. If the trough level indicates that the drug is present in subtherapeutic levels, the drug dosage will be increased to be therapeutic.

tuberculin syringe or TB syringe. A small syringe often manufactured with a 25-gauge needle, the tuberculin syringe can only hold a total of one milliliter. It is used for the Mantoux test for tuberculosis, hence its name. It is also used for measuring pediatric injections.

vasodilator A drug that relaxes the smooth muscle of blood vessels to improve blood flow.

vasopressor A drug that constricts smooth muscle of blood vessels to increase blood pressure.

vial A small glass bottle containing a liquid or powder for injection. It has a rubber stopper in the cap which allows for injection of diluent for reconstitution of the powder. The rubber stopper also allows repeated doses of the drug to be withdrawn from the same vial.

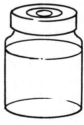

FIGURE 8-2

Vial

9

Systems of Measurement

In the early history of pharmacology, measurements of drug dosages were crude and imprecise. The powdered, dried herbs in many prescriptions contained varying amounts of active drug which could not be measured.

Apothecary System

In the 1700s, the apothecary system was introduced from England. The term *apothecary* comes from a Greek word and refers to a person who combines and dispenses drugs. Some apothecary measurements are still in use today. These include the liquid measurements of pint, quart, and gallon. Apothecary measurements for calculating liquid doses of drugs included the minim, grain, scruple, and dram. (The standard of a grain was originally based on the average weight of one grain of wheat.) In past years the apothecary measurements of minim, scruple, and dram have fallen into disuse. Today, most drug dosages are measured by the metric system. The apothecary measurement of a grain does have limited use, however. A few drugs (phenobarbital, for example) are manufactured in equivalent apothecary and metric doses, such as 1/2 grain and 30 milligrams.

Metric System

The metric system was invented by the French in 1790. It is based on the length of a meter which was originally calculated by dividing the earth's circumference by 10 million. The use of the metric system was made legal but not mandatory in the United States in 1866. In 1975 Congress passed the Metric Conversion Act, but with the exception of scientists, doctors, and other professionals in scientific fields, few laypersons use the metric system on a regular basis. However, nearly all of the drugs manufactured use doses based on the metric system.

The metric system is officially known as the International System of Units (SI). The SI was officially adopted as the exclusive unit of measurement by the American Medical Association on July 1, 1988, although some reference books do not reflect this change. The SI metric system is based on the kilogram (for weight measurements), the liter (for volume measurements), and the meter (for length measurements). Metric weight measurements include the kilogram, gram, milligram, and microgram. Each of these differs by a factor of 1000.

1 kilogram = 1000 grams (*khilioi* is Greek for *one thousand*)
1 gram = 1000 milligrams (*mille* is Latin for *one thousand*)
1 milligram = 1000 micrograms
(*Mikros* is Greek for *small* and stands for *one million*.
A microgram is one-millionth of a gram.)

Drug weight measurements are not expressed in terms of kilograms, which are more appropriately used to describe a person's weight. (Example: A 110-pound woman weighs 50 kilograms.) Extremely premature infants may be measured in grams. (Example: A 900-gram premature infant weighs just under 2 pounds.) Most drugs are measured not in grams but in milligrams and occasionally in micrograms.

The metric system also includes the liquid measurements of liter and milliliter. Drugs are not prescribed by the liter; the milliliter (mL) is used frequently, however.

1 liter = 1000 milliliters

For example, a common dose for the antacid Maalox is 30 mL. The Mantoux intradermal test for tuberculosis involves the injection of 0.1 mL of solution.

The basic measurement of length in the metric system is the meter. The centimeter is equivalent to 1/100 of a meter. When a cube is formed that is one centimeter long on each side, it becomes a measurement of volume known as the cubic centimeter. This volume measurement is equivalent to the volume contained in a milliliter, and the two volume abbreviations *mL* and *cc* are used interchangeably.

Common abbreviations for metric measurements are as follows.

cubic centimeter	cc
kilogram	kg
gram	g (not *gm*, which is obsolete)
	(not *gr.*, which is the abbreviation for *grain*)
milligram	mg
microgram	mcg
milliliter	mL

Note: Metric abbreviations are not followed by a period. The abbreviation for grain (gr.) is followed by a period because it is from the apothecary system.

Other types of drug dosage measurements include unit, inch, drop, milliequivalent, percentage, ratio, household.

1. **Unit.** The dosages of certain drugs are never measured by the metric system but by a special designation called a unit. Some penicillins, some vitamins, and all types of insulin are measured in units. The exact value of a unit varies from drug to drug. A unit of penicillin was standardized in 1944 as 0.6 mcg of penicillin G based on its ability to cause a ring of inhibition of a certain size on a bacterial culture. Other types of penicillin are measured in milligrams. The International Unit (IU) is used to measure the fat soluble vitamins A, D, and E. Other vitamins are measured in milligrams. All forms of insulin are measured in units. The unit of insulin is defined on the weight basis of pure insulin with 28 units equaling one milligram. Insulin is manufactured in solutions with 100 units per milliliter, abbreviated as U-100.

2. **Inch.** Only one commonly prescribed drug is measured in inches, and that is nitroglycerin ointment. Special applicator papers are supplied with each tube of ointment for the purpose of accurately measuring the dose. The ointment is squeezed onto the applicator paper along the marking lines in 1/2 inch increments. The dose may range from 1/2 inch to 2 inches or more. The paper is then applied to the skin and taped.

3. **Drop.** The Latin word for *drops* is *guttae*; the abbreviation for drops is *gtt.* Eye and ear liquid medications are often prescribed in the number of drops to be given.

4. **Milliequivalent.** An equivalent is the molecular weight of an ion divided by the number of hydrogen ions it reacts with. This number is expressed in grams. A milliequivalent (mEq) is 1/1000 of an equivalent. Doses of electrolytes, such as potassium which is an ion, are measured in milliequivalents, although their doses can also be given in milligrams.

5. **Percentage.** A percentage is one part in relationship to the whole, based on a total of 100. Thus a 10% solution would be composed of one gram of drug in 10 milliliters of solution. A 1% preparation of the steroid ointment triamcinolone (Aristocort, Kenalog), would contain 1 mg of drug in 100 mg of white petrolatum base.

6. **Ratio.** A ratio expresses the relationship between the concentrations of two substances together in solution. A ratio is expressed as two numbers with a colon mark between. Example: Epinephrine for intracardiac injection during resuscitation is supplied in a ratio of 1:10,000 (or one part epinephrine to 10,000 parts of solution). Epinephrine for subcutaneous injection with a local anesthetic is supplied in a ratio of 1:100,000.

7. **Household measurement.** The household system of measurement is an unofficial system that patients use in their homes for measuring drugs. It includes everyday teaspoons and tablespoons. This is an inaccurate measurement system because there is no standard size for teaspoons and tablespoons. In fact, a teaspoon can hold anywhere from 4 to 7 mL of liquid. Many over-the-counter medicines (cough syrup, for example) have instructions on the label to measure the dose in teaspoons but include a standardized plastic medicine cup with measured teaspoon markings to ensure proper dosing.

Number Forms

The apothecary system uses fractions to express dosages less than one (example: phenobarbital gr. 1/4).

Measurements in the metric system are never expressed in fractions. Metric numbers less than one are written as decimals, such as 0.125 mg. The decimal point must be placed carefully; an error in placement can mean a 10-fold increase or decrease in the drug dose. Metric numbers less than one always have a zero added to the left of the decimal point (example: 0.5 mg, not .5 mg).

Roman numerals were often used with the old apothecary measurements. Today, however, Roman numerals are used in handwritten prescriptions for medications which are given by drops and occasionally for those given by capsule or tablet, at the discretion of the physician writing the prescription. The Roman numeral is not written in standard form as I, II, III, or IV, but is handwritten in the following way.

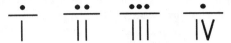

Note: These symbols do not represent fractions although they do resemble them to some extent. A typewriter cannot reproduce these symbols, so an Arabic number is used in place of these modified Roman numerals.

Some numbers written after a drug name are an integral part of the drug's name and do not indicate the amount of the drug to be taken.

Maalox II (a double-strength formula of regular Maalox)

Tylenol No. 3 (a combination drug containing 300 mg of Tylenol and 30 mg of codeine)

Dosage Schedules

Drugs are measured not only in terms of the amount of the dosage but also in terms of the frequency of the dosage. There are a number of commonly used abbreviations which indicate the frequency of administration. These abbreviations are based on Latin words, as indicated.

Abbreviation	Latin	Medical Meaning
a.c.	ante cibum	before meals
ad lib.	ad libitum	as needed
b.i.d.	bis in die	twice a day
c̄	cum	with
h.s.	hora somni	at bedtime (hour of sleep)
n.p.o.	nihil per os	nothing by mouth
p.c.	post cibum	after meals
p.r.n.	pro re nata	as needed
q.d.	quaque die	every day
q.h.	quaque hora	every hour
q.h.s.	quaque hora somni	every bedtime
q.i.d.	quater in die	four times a day
q.o.d.	(informal usage)	every other day
s̄	sine	without
t.i.d.	ter in die	three times a day

Dosage Calculations

The standard adult dose for a drug is appropriate for most adults and is calculated to encompass a range appropriate to the size and age of most patients. Patients who are elderly, extremely thin, or extremely obese may have their drug dosage adjusted.

Pediatric doses, especially those for infants and prematures, must be calculated with great accuracy. Doses calculated on the basis of age alone cannot be individually tailored to each child. Therefore, the pediatric drug dose is usually calculated individually based on the total body weight for each patient, not according to age. Because the weight of a pediatric patient may change rapidly, these calculations are periodically adjusted. Pediatric drug doses are expressed as **mg/kg/day** or milligrams of drug needed per kilogram of body weight per 24-hour period.

Chemotherapy drugs are specially calculated using the patient's total body surface area. Doses are expressed in milligrams per meter squared (**mg/m²**).

REVIEW QUESTIONS

1. What is the only apothecary measurement for drugs still in use today?
2. Name three metric measurements used to weigh drugs.
3. A milliliter is equivalent to a cubic centimeter in volume. True or False?
4. Give the definition of these common abbreviations:
   a.c.
   b.i.d.
   g
   gr.
   h.s.
   mcg
   mg
   mL
   mEq
   p.r.n.
   q.i.d.
   t.i.d.
5. Name three drugs measured in units.
6. Name one drug measured in inches.
7. Pediatric drug doses are individually calculated on the basis of what criteria?

SPELLING TIPS

- milliequivalent (often mispronounced as "millequivalent"). The abbreviation *mEq* is unusual for its internal capitalization.

10

The Prescription

The term *prescription* comes from the Latin word *praescriptio,* meaning *a written order.* A prescription is the written record of a physician's order for the pharmacist to dispense medication to a patient.

By law, all drugs are classified as either prescription or nonprescription. Prescription drugs can be ordered only by a physician or a dentist. Prescriptions are usually imprinted with the physician's name and address.

IMA N. PAINE, M.D.
2105 Lancey Dr., Suite 1, Modesto, CA 95355
Phone (209) 551-2114

Name _____   Date _____

Address _____

R_x

_____ M.D.

FIGURE 10-1
Typical prescription form

Prescription drugs with a potential for abuse or physical/psychological dependence (i.e., schedule drugs or controlled drugs) are further restricted under the Controlled Substances Act of 1970. For schedule drugs, the physician's assigned DEA (Drug Enforcement Administration) number must be included for the prescription to be valid.

Each prescription is composed of several parts as described below.

1. **Rx.** This symbol stands for the Latin word *recipe,* meaning *take.* Prescriptions were, at one time, actually recipes listing several ingredients to be mixed by the pharmacist before dispensing. Most prescription pads come with a large preprinted Rx just to the left of the area where the prescription itself will be handwritten.

2. **Drug name.** The drug name may be a generic or trade name. The chemical name of a drug is seldom used in writing a prescription (exceptions: ferrous sulfate, zinc oxide).

3. **Drug strength.** The first number after the drug name may indicate the amount of drug per tablet. Later in the prescription after *Sig.*, the number of tablets to be taken at each dose is indicated.

4. **#.** This symbol is read as *number* and indicates to the pharmacist the total number of capsules, tablets, or ounces of drug to dispense to the patient. Sometimes the physician will preface the number sign with the abbreviation for the word *dispense* (example: Disp. #30). The total number of tablets, etc., is based on the estimated length of treatment and how many are to be taken each day.

5. **Sig.** This abbreviation stands for the Latin word *signetur,* meaning *write on the label.* It indicates that the instructions for the use of the drug will follow (example: Sig.: 2 caps). These instructions, which tell the patient the amount and frequency of the dose, are also written on the patient's prescription bottle by the pharmacist. Sometimes the abbreviation *Sig.* is not written on the prescription, and the drug name is followed directly by numbers indicating the amount and frequency of the dose. This is especially true when the drug is manufactured in only one strength.

6. **Frequency.** The frequency includes how often the dose is to be administered. This is usually written as a Latin abbreviation describing how many times a day or at what time of day the drug should be taken (example: b.i.d. or h.s.).

7. **Route of administration.** This indicates whether the drug is to be given orally, topically, vaginally, intravenously, etc. Most routes of administration are expressed as an abbreviation derived from Latin words. (Example: *PO* or *p.o.* stands for *per os* which means *by mouth.*)

8. **Refills.** The physician indicates how many times the patient is permitted to refill the prescription before being reevaluated medically. On some prescription forms, there is a preprinted box which says *refills*, followed by the numbers 1, 2, and 3. The physician simply circles the appropriate number to indicate how many refills are indicated. Refills may also be written in this way: Refills x 2. Refills of schedule drugs are limited by law.

9. **Signature line.** At the bottom of the prescription form, there is a preprinted line with M.D. at the far right-hand side. The physician must sign his or her name in order for the prescription to be valid even if the name and address are preprinted at the top of the prescription blank.

10. **DEA number.** If a schedule drug is prescribed, the physician is required by law to also write in his or her DEA number.

Other information that is usually preprinted on prescription forms includes the doctor's name and address, a space for the patient's name and address, and a space for the date the prescription is written.

In the hospital, the physician orders, renews, or discontinues drugs by writing the prescription on the physician's order sheet at the front of the patient's chart. The order sheet contains several carbon copies, one of which is removed every time a new order is written and sent to the hospital pharmacy where the drug is dispensed or discontinued.

11

Dermatology Drugs

Because of the superficial nature and location of most dermatologic diseases, they respond well to topical drug therapy. Mild cases of skin diseases such as acne, psoriasis, poison ivy, contact dermatitis, superficial infections, herpes simplex infections, lice, and diaper rash can be successfully treated with topical agents. However, drugs which act systemically may be necessary when dermatologic diseases become widespread or particularly severe. For example, a variety of over-the-counter products are effective in providing relief from mild, localized cases of poison ivy. However, a widespread case with large areas of open, weeping lesions is difficult to treat with topical medication. A prescription-strength drug may be indicated for relief of symptoms; an oral steroid or antihistamine might be prescribed to relieve inflammation and severe itching.

This chapter will describe common over-the-counter and prescription drugs used topically to treat dermatologic diseases.

Acne Drugs

Various creams, lotions, and gels are used topically to cleanse away oil and dead skin (keratolytic action), to close the pores (astringent action), to inhibit the growth of skin bacteria (antiseptic action), and to kill skin bacteria (antibiotic action). The over-the-counter products listed below are used to treat acne vulgaris, the acne common in adolescence:

> benzoyl peroxide
> Clearasil
> Fostex
> Oxy 5, Oxy 10
> Propa P.H.
> Stri-Dex

Prescription antibiotics may be used topically to treat more serious cases of acne vulgaris. These include:

> Benzamycin (a combination of erythromycin and benzoyl peroxide)
> clindamycin (Cleocin T)
> erythromycin (Eryderm, Staticin)
> meclocycline (Meclan)
> tetracycline (Topicycline)

51

Tetracycline may also be prescribed orally for systemic treatment of acne vulgaris.

Severe cystic acne which may be unresponsive to antibiotic treatment may be treated with topical tretinoin (Retin-A), a form of vitamin A. It causes skin cells to multiply more rapidly. This rapid turnover prevents pores from becoming clogged and infected. A structurally related drug, isotretinoin (Accutane), is prescribed orally for the same purpose.

Acne rosacea, an adult form of acne not caused by excessive oil but exacerbated by heat, stress, and skin irritation, is treated with metronidazole (MetroGel).

Psoriasis Drugs

Various topical agents are used to treat psoriasis. Among them are **coal tar** lotions, gels, and shampoos that cleanse away dead skin (keratolytic action) and decrease itching (antipruritic action). These trade name products include Balnetar, Denorex, Estar, Tegrin, and Zetar. Other drugs used to treat psoriasis include the topical corticosteroids, discussed in the next section.

> DID YOU KNOW? Coal tar, a byproduct of the processing of bituminous coal, contains over 10,000 different chemical ingredients. It has been used since the 1800s to treat psoriasis.

Systemic drugs are used to treat severe psoriasis uncontrolled by topical agents. These include etretinate (Tegison) and methotrexate (Folex). Note: Methotrexate is a well-known chemotherapy agent which acts by inhibiting DNA synthesis. This action is most effective in rapidly dividing cells such as cancer cells. When used to treat psoriasis, it is effective because psoriatic skin cells have been found to divide at a much faster rate than normal skin cells.

Severe, disabling psoriasis, unresponsive to any of the above drugs, may be treated with methoxsalen (Oxsoralen). This is used only in conjunction with exposure to ultraviolet light. The drug sensitizes the skin to the effects of ultraviolet light; the ultraviolet light damages cell DNA and decreases rates of cell division. Methoxsalen belongs to a group of drugs known as **psoralens.** The combination therapy of methoxsalen and ultraviolet light is known as **PUVA** (psoralen/ultraviolet wavelength A).

Topical Corticosteroids

Steroid is a general term encompassing a number of hormones produced by the body. *Corticosteroids* comprise those produced by the adrenal gland. Within this large group, there are corticosteroids which act to suppress the immune system's response to tissue damage. These corticosteroids are used to decrease tissue inflammation and itching. Hydrocortisone, introduced in 1952, was the first topical corticosteroid. In 1983, it was also the first approved in a nonprescription strength for over-the-counter sales. Topical corticosteroids, both over-the-counter and prescription, are indicated for the relief of contact dermatitis, poison ivy, insect bites, and to treat psoriasis, seborrhea, and eczema. Oral corticosteroids may be given to act systemically in cases of severe inflammation or itching. (See page 108.)

Topical corticosteroids come in several strengths as indicated by a percentage following the trade name. Some common over-the-counter and prescription generic and trade name topical corticosteroid agents include:

      amcinonide (Cyclocort)
      betamethasone (Diprosone, Uticort, Valisone)
      clocortolone (Cloderm)
      desonide (Tridesilon)
      desoximetasone (Topicort)
      dexamethasone (Decaderm, Decadron)
      fluocinolone (Lidex, Synalar)
      flurandrenolide (Cordran)
      halcinonide (Halog)
      hydrocortisone (CaldeCort, Cortaid, Cortef, Cortril, Hycort, Hytone)
      triamcinolone (Aristocort, Kenalog)

Note: The endings -*sone, -olone,* and -*onide* are common to some generic corticosteroids.

Topical Antibiotics

Antibiotics are used topically to treat minor skin infections. They act by inhibiting or killing bacteria by blocking their ability to maintain a cell wall. Topical antibiotics are manufactured as gels, lotions, creams, ointments, and sprays. Common generic and trade name topical antibiotics include:

      bacitracin
      chloramphenicol (Chloromycetin)
      erythromycin
      gentamicin (Garamycin)
      neomycin
      oxytetracycline (Terramycin)
      tetracycline (Achromycin)

DID YOU KNOW? Bacitracin is used only topically because it can produce toxic effects when given systemically. It was developed from a strain of bacteria found growing in a culture of wound drainage from a patient named Margaret Tracy. The name *bacitracin* is a combination of the names of the bacteria and the patient, *Bacillus subtilis* and *Tracy.*

Some products combine several antibiotics together.

      Bactine antibiotic ointment (bacitracin, neomycin, and polymyxin B)
      Neosporin (bacitracin and polymyxin B)
      Polysporin (bacitracin and polymyxin B)

Topical corticosteroid and antibiotic drugs are often combined to form combination products such as:

Cordran-N (hydrocortisone and neomycin)
Cortisporin (hydrocortisone, polymyxin B, and neomycin)

Topical Antifungals

Fungus infections such as ringworm (tinea corporis), athlete's foot (tinea pedis), and jock itch (tinea cruris) can be effectively treated with topical antifungal drugs. These drugs alter the cell wall of the fungus and disrupt enzyme activity, resulting in cell death. These over-the-counter and prescription drugs are manufactured in topical cream, ointment, and powder forms, and include:

over-the-counter
Desenex
miconazole (Micatin)
tolnaftate (Tinactin)
prescription
ciclopirox (Loprox)
clotrimazole (Lotrimin, Mycelex)
econazole (Spectazole)
haloprogin (Halotex)
ketoconazole (Nizoral)
naftifine (Naftin)
oxiconazole (Oxistat)
sulconazole (Exelderm)

Note: The ending *-azole* is common to many generic antifungal drugs.

When topical fungal infections are severe, become embedded in the nails (onychomycosis), or become systemic, ketoconazole (Nizoral), griseofulvin (Grifulvin), or fluconazole (Diflucan) may be given orally, or fluconazole or amphotericin B (Fungizone) may be given intravenously. See also Chapter 29.

Yeasts are closely related to fungi. See Chapter 19 for drugs used to treat oral yeast infections; see Chapter 23 for drugs used to treat vaginal yeast infections.

Antiviral Drugs

Herpes simplex virus type 2 infections involve the genital area while type 1 infections involve other areas of the body, particularly the mouth. These painful and infectious lesions are treated topically with acyclovir (Zovirax). They may also be treated with intralesional injections of

interferon alfa-2b (Intron A)
interferon alfa-n3 (Alferon N)

The severe pain of herpes zoster virus infections, also known as shingles, is treated topically with capsaicin (Zostrix), a derivative of red pepper.

Topical Antihistamines

While corticosteroids inhibit inflammation regardless of its source, antihistamines only inhibit inflammation, redness, and itching caused by an allergic reaction and the release of histamine, hence the name *antihistamines*. Common topical antihistamines include diphenhydramine (Benadryl) and the combination product Caladryl (diphenhydramine and calamine). For severe itching, antihistamines such as diphenhydramine (Benadryl) or cyproheptadine (Periactin) may be given orally, or the anti-anxiety drug hydroxyzine (Vistaril, Atarax) may be given.

All drugs which relieve itching topically or systemically are known as **antipruritics**. (*Pruritus* means *itching.*)

Topical Anesthetics
See Chapter 31, page 156.

Drugs for Scabies and Lice
Scabies is caused by mites, tiny parasites which tunnel under the skin causing itchy lesions. The prescription drug lindane (Kwell), applied to the body as a lotion, is curative. (The head is rarely infected.) Scabies in humans is caused by the same parasite which causes mange in dogs.

Pediculosis, an infestation of lice, is found on both the head and body. Lice are easily transmitted on combs and hats among school children. Nonprescription treatments such as RID and Triple X contain the active ingredient pyrethrin which is derived from chrysanthemums. It acts on the nervous system of the parasite to paralyze it. Pyrethrin is a common ingredient in flea powder as well. Prescription drugs used to treat lice include lindane (Kwell), R & C, and permethrin (Nix). The last two drugs contain a synthetic pyrethrin.

DID YOU KNOW? The term *nit-picking,* meaning *to point out and criticize tiny details*, comes from the process of picking through the hair looking for lice eggs which are called *nits.*

Miscellaneous Dermatologic Drugs

A and D An ointment containing vitamins A and D to promote healing.

AgNO₃ See *silver nitrate.*

Aveeno An oatmeal and lanolin solution used as a lotion or in bath water to treat the itching and weeping lesions of poison ivy, chickenpox, and hives.

Betadine An orange-brown antibiotic soap used as a hand scrub prior to surgery and as a solution painted on an operative site. Also available as an ointment, often placed around I.V. line and catheter entry sites. The active ingredient is iodine.

Burow's solution Applied as a wet dressing to relieve superficial inflammation from insect bites, poison ivy, and athlete's foot. Not a trade name drug; named for Dr. Karl August von Burow, the German surgeon.

calamine A lotion used for poison ivy, insect bites, and sunburn, it decreases itching and soothes.

Desitin An ointment for diaper rash, it contains zinc oxide to coat and protect, and cod liver oil with vitamin A to promote healing.

Domeboro   A trade name tablet or powder which, when mixed with water, produces Burow's solution. See *Burow's solution.*

gentian violet   An antibacterial and antifungal agent. This deep purple solution is sometimes used prophylactically on the umbilical cords of newborns. This drug is also known as **triple dye** because it contains three different purple dyes which are the active drug ingredients.

Hibiclens   An antibacterial scrub and skin cleaner.

mafenide (Sulfamylon)   An agent which inhibits bacterial growth, it is applied to second- and third-degree burns to prevent infection.

minoxidil (Rogaine)   Used to treat male pattern baldness, minoxidil dilates arteries in the scalp which stimulates hair growth in some patients. Note: Minoxidil is also used to treat hypertension and is marketed for that purpose under the trade names Loniten and Minodyl.

Mycolog-II   Combination of triamcinolone and nystatin.

nitrofurazone (Furacin)   An antibiotic applied specifically to second- and third-degree burns to prevent infection.

pHisoHex   This antibacterial skin scrub generated controversy some years ago when it was found to cause seizures when applied to newborns with diaper rash. (The hexachlorophene in it was absorbed through broken skin into the bloodstream.) It is no longer administered that way. A similar product, pHisoDerm, contains no hexachlorophene and has no antibacterial properties.

silver nitrate (chemical name $AgNO_3$)   Topical antiseptic with caustic qualities. Used to seal and cauterize small bleeding areas in the nose during epistaxis, to remove skin lesions nonsurgically in podiatry, and on the umbilical cord as a topical antiseptic.

silver sulfadiazine (Silvadene)   An antibiotic applied specifically to second- and third-degree burns to prevent infection. The active component is silver ions.

tretinoin (Retin-A)   The same drug (discussed earlier) which is used to treat acne vulgaris is also used topically to decrease wrinkle lines on the face, particularly around the eyes.

triple dye   See *gentian violet.*

zinc oxide   Used topically for skin irritation and diaper rash to coat and protect.

REVIEW QUESTIONS

1. Explain why some dermatologic diseases (such as poison ivy) may be treated with either topical or systemic drugs.
2. How does the anti-inflammatory and antipruritic action of an antihistamine differ from that of a corticosteroid? Why is it not appropriate to treat all kinds of itching dermatological diseases with an antihistamine?
3. Coal tar preparations and psoralens are prescribed for what dermatologic disease?
4. The drug minoxidil is used to treat both hypertension and male pattern baldness. True or False?

12

Urinary Tract Drugs

Urinary tract drugs include diuretics (used to treat hypertension), urinary tract antibiotics and other anti-infection agents, urinary tract analgesics, urinary antispasmodics, and potassium supplements taken concurrently with many diuretics to counteract their potassium-wasting effect.

Diuretics

The kidneys filter circulating blood, extracting waste products, water, sodium, potassium, and various other substances. They also regulate the blood volume by retaining or excreting sodium ions which in turn cause water to be retained or excreted. Diuretics increase the natural excretion of sodium (and therefore also water). By causing extra sodium and water to be excreted from the circulating blood volume, diuretics are useful in the treatment of hypertension.

Diuretics are divided into several groups on the basis of their action within the nephron of the kidney: thiazide diuretics, loop diuretics, and potassium-sparing diuretics.

Thiazide diuretics act at the site of the distal renal tubule within the nephron. They increase the excretion of sodium (and therefore water) in the urine. The thiazide diuretics include:

   bendroflumethiazide (Naturetin)
   chlorothiazide (Diuril)
   hydrochlorothiazide (abbreviated HCTZ) (Esidrix, HydroDIURIL, Oretic)
   hydroflumethiazide (Diucardin, Saluron)
   methyclothiazide (Enduron)
   polythiazide (Renese)
   quinethazone (Hydromox)
   trichlormethiazide (Diurese)

Note: The ending *-iazide* is common to generic thiazide diuretics.

   Other diuretics closely related in structure and action to the thiazide diuretics are:

   chlorthalidone (Hygroton)
   metolazone (Zaroxolyn)

Loop diuretics act at the site of the proximal and distal tubules as well as the loop of Henle (hence their name). They block the reabsorption of sodium into the bloodstream so that it is excreted along with water into the urine. The loop diuretics include:

> bumetanide (Bumex)
> ethacrynic acid (Edecrin)
> furosemide (Lasix)

Both thiazide and loop diuretics cause sodium and water to be excreted. Sodium is a positive ion (Na^+). The action of these diuretics also causes potassium, another positive ion (K^+), to be excreted. The excessive loss of potassium can cause serious side effects, including cardiac arrhythmias. Patients who need to take a thiazide or loop diuretic may also be given potassium supplements, or they may take a potassium-sparing diuretic alone or in combination with the other diuretics to offset the potassium-wasting effect.

The **potassium-sparing diuretics** include:

> amiloride (Midamor)
> spironolactone (Aldactone)
> triamterene (Dyrenium)

Some products combine a thiazide diuretic with a potassium-sparing diuretic in one tablet. These combination products include:

> Aldactazide (hydrochlorothiazide and spironolactone)
> Dyazide (hydrochlorothiazide and triamterene)
> Maxzide (hydrochlorothiazide and triamterene)
> Moduretic (hydrochlorothiazide and amiloride)

The diuretic mannitol (Osmitrol) is used only in cases of impending renal failure to stimulate the production of urine, and to relieve cerebral edema and decrease intracranial pressure. It is given intravenously only.

Potassium Supplements

Potassium supplements are frequently prescribed for patients taking thiazide and loop diuretics to avoid potassium depletion. Although some foods, such as bananas, are rich in potassium, dietary sources alone are usually not sufficient to replenish potassium loss from diuretics. Potassium supplements are manufactured as liquids (patients often object to the taste), powders and effervescent tablets to be mixed with water, capsules, and tablets. Dosages are measured in milliequivalents (mEq). Trade name potassium supplements include:

> Kay Ciel
> K-Dur
> K-Lor
> Klorvess
> Klotrix
> K-Lyte
> K-Tab
> Micro-K
> Potage
> Slow-K

Note: The presence of *K* in nearly every trade name for potassium supplements refers to the chemical symbol for potassium (K^+).

Drugs for Urinary Tract Infections

Urinary tract infections are often treated with oral antibiotics which exert a systemic effect, particularly those effective against gram-negative *E. coli,* a contaminating pathogen from the GI tract. (See Chapter 27.) However, urinary tract infections can also be treated with special urinary tract antibiotics which, while given orally, do not exert a systemic effect but concentrate in the renal tubules to kill bacteria. These drugs include:

> cinoxacin (Cinobac)
> nalidixic acid (NegGram)
> nitrofurantoin (Furadantin, Macrodantin)
> norfloxacin (Noroxin)

Note: The trade name NegGram was selected because the drug is effective against gram-negative bacteria, the primary cause of urinary tract infections.

Another drug used for urinary tract infections is methenamine (Hiprex, Mandelamine). It is not an antibiotic, but in the urine it is changed to ammonia and formaldehyde which exert a direct effect, killing bacteria.

Urinary tract infections can also be treated with **sulfonamides.** These drugs are not true antibiotics because they only inhibit the growth of bacteria but do not kill them in the way antibiotics do. The sulfonamides (also called *sulfa drugs*) include:

> sulfacytine (Renoquid)
> sulfamethizole (Thiosulfil Forte)
> sulfamethoxazole (Gantanol)
> sulfisoxazole (Gantrisin)
> triple sulfa (Neotrizine, Terfonyl)

Urinary Tract Analgesics

Urinary tract infections and other diseases have associated symptoms of burning and frequent, painful urination. Urinary tract analgesics exert a topical pain-relieving effect only on the mucosa of the urinary tract, even though these drugs are given orally. The most common urinary tract analgesic is phenazopyridine (Pyridium, Urogesic).

Pyridium Plus is a trade name combination drug which contains a urinary analgesic, an antispasmodic, and a sedative.

The trade name drug Azo Gantrisin combines a sulfonamide for its anti-infection action and a urinary tract analgesic for control of pain.

Urinary Antispasmodics and Cholinergics

Irritation in the urinary tract from infection, catheterization, urinary retention, or kidney stones can result in ureteral spasms, renal colic, or spasm of the bladder sphincter. Antispasmodic drugs used to treat these symptoms include:

> flavoxate (Urispas)
> L-hyoscyamine (Anaspaz, Cystospaz).

A cholinergic drug used to treat these same symptoms, which acts by stimulating cholinergic receptors in the smooth muscle of the bladder to contract, is bethanechol (Duvoid, Urecholine).

Miscellaneous Drugs

epoetin alfa (Epogen)   A protein, manufactured by recombinant DNA techniques, which stimulates the production of red blood cells. This drug is used to treat patients in chronic renal failure who have anemia.

REVIEW QUESTIONS

1. Describe the therapeutic action of diuretics and how it is useful for treating hypertension.
2. What is the difference between a thiazide diuretic and a loop diuretic?
3. Why do so many potassium supplements contain the capital letter *K* in the trade name?
4. What is the meaning of the abbreviation *HCTZ*?

SPELLING TIPS

- Dyazide (Spelled *Dy*, not *Di*.)
- NegGram (Unusual for its internal capitalization.)
- HydroDIURIL (Unusual use of all capital letters for the second part of the drug.)
- Kay Ciel (When dictated, it is often not recognized as a trade name, but is mistakenly transcribed as *KCl*, an abbreviation of the chemical name *potassium chloride.*)
- Urispas, Anaspaz, Cystospaz (Similar sounding trade names ending in different letters.)

13

Gastrointestinal Drugs

Gastrointestinal drugs are prescribed to treat disease conditions of the stomach and intestines such as ulcers, diarrhea, constipation, ulcerative colitis, irritable bowel syndrome, or gallstones.

Ulcer Drugs

Peptic ulcer is a general term used to describe ulcers in the esophagus, stomach or duodenum. A gastric ulcer is located in the stomach. All peptic ulcers are caused by irritation of the mucous membrane of the gastrointestinal tract from the hypersecretion of hydrochloric acid and the subsequent action of pepsin which digests protein. Aspirin, nonsteroidal anti-inflammatory drugs (NSAID), alcohol, and caffeine also irritate the mucous membranes and can contribute to ulcer formation. Several types of drugs are used to treat ulcers. These include antacids, H_2 blockers, antispasmodics, and others.

Antacids

Antacids were the original, and for many years the only, treatment for peptic ulcers. They are weak bases which exert a therapeutic effect by neutralizing acid. By raising the pH, they also inhibit the action of pepsin. They contain aluminum, magnesium, calcium, sodium, or a combination of these as the active ingredients. Antacids are available without a prescription.

Antacids containing aluminum as the active ingredient include:
Alternagel
Amphojel
Basaljel
Antacids containing magnesium as the active ingredient include milk of magnesia.
Antacids containing a combination of aluminum and magnesium include:
Di-Gel
Gelusil
Maalox, Maalox II
Mylanta
Riopan
Antacids containing calcium as the active ingredient include:
Rolaids
Titralac
Tums

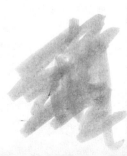

61

The use of calcium-containing antacids can have an additional benefit for women by supplementing dietary calcium intake.

Antacids containing sodium as the active ingredient include:

Alka-Seltzer

baking soda

Bromo Seltzer

Although sodium bicarbonate neutralizes acid, it is not recommended as a long-term treatment for ulcers because of the large amount of sodium absorbed systemically. Physicians recommend the prudent use of salt (sodium) even for patients without hypertension and other medical conditions.

DID YOU KNOW? One dose of regular Alka-Seltzer contains 958 mg of sodium. For patients on a low-salt diet, one dose could equal their recommended allowance of sodium for the entire day.

Note: Although antacids have an anti-acid effect, the *i* is omitted from *anti* in the correct spelling of this class of drugs.

Some antacids contain an additional ingredient to relieve flatulence. Simethicone acts by changing the surface tension of air bubbles trapped in the GI tract to allow them to be expelled. Antacids which contain simethicone include:

Di-Gel

Gelusil

Maalox Plus

Mylanta

Simethicone is also available alone under the trade names of:

Gas-X

Mylicon

Phazyme

These drugs have no antacid action, however.

H₂ Blockers

The release of gastric acid is triggered by histamine which acts on special histamine receptors (known as H_2 receptors) in the gastric parietal cells lining the stomach. Drugs which block these receptors and prevent the release of acid are known as H_2 blockers and are used to treat ulcers.

H_2 blockers currently prescribed to treat ulcers include:

cimetidine (Tagamet)

famotidine (Pepcid)

nizatidine (Axid)

ranitidine (Zantac)

Note: The ending *-tidine* is common in the generic name of H_2 blockers.

HISTORICAL NOTE: The effects of antihistamines have been known since diphenhydramine (Benadryl) was introduced in 1946. It was known that histamine was released in response to allergic reactions (causing red, itching eyes and a runny nose) and that antihistamine drugs could prevent these symptoms. It was also known that histamine was released in the stomach to stimulate the production of acid. This release of histamine was not related to an allergic reaction and could not be prevented by antihistamine drugs. Therefore it was postulated that histamine acted upon two different receptors, designated as H_1 and H_2 receptors.

Researchers at Smith, Kline & French pharmaceutical company began to search for a drug that could block the action of histamine on H_2 receptors in the stomach. Such a drug would prevent the release of acid and would be useful in the treatment of ulcers. By rearranging the chemical structure of a molecule of histamine, they developed a drug which would combine with H_2 receptors but would not actually activate them, thus effectively "blocking" both the receptors and the release of acid. This type of drug which "blocks" a receptor is generally referred to as an antagonist. The new drug was the first of the H_2 blockers and was named cimetidine. For the trade name, Smith, Kline & French combined syllables from **ant**agonist and **cimet**idine to make Tagamet, released in 1979.

Other Ulcer Drugs

misoprostol (Cytotec)   Given to patients on long-term aspirin or nonsteroidal antiinflammatory drugs (NSAID) to prevent their common side effect of gastric ulcers. Aspirin and NSAIDs inhibit the formation of prostaglandins; prostaglandins produce inflammation and pain in arthritis, but also normally act to protect the gastric mucosa. Misoprostol is a synthetic prostaglandin which protects the gastric mucosa when natural prostaglandin is inhibited by arthritis drugs.

pirenzepine (Gastrozepine)   An investigational anti-ulcer drug similar in its effect to that of cimetidine, although it is not an H_2 blocker.

A unique anti-ulcer drug unrelated to either antacids or H_2 blockers is **sucralfate (Carafate).** This drug acts topically on the ulcer surface. It is attracted to injured areas of the mucous membrane which are draining fluid high in protein. The drug binds directly to these areas, forming a protective layer or bandage over the ulcer, allowing it to heal.

Antispasmodics

Intestinal conditions such as irritable bowel syndrome, spastic colon, diverticulitis, and even ulcers can be accompanied by abdominal pain due to spasms. These spasms can be relieved by a category of drugs known as **anticholinergics** which decrease spasms by slowing peristalsis, the rhythmic waves of contractions which propel food through the GI tract.

Anticholinergics exert their therapeutic action in the following way. Motility and peristalsis in the gastrointestinal tract are controlled by the parasympathetic nervous system through the release of the neurotransmitter acetylcholine. Acetylcholine then acts on cholinergic receptors in the gastrointestinal tract to begin peristalsis. If peristalsis is too strong due to the disease conditions mentioned above, anticholinergic drugs can be given which block the effects of acetylcholine on cholinergic receptors.

Anticholinergic drugs used as antispasmodics include:

anisotropine (Valpin)
clidinium (Quarzan)
dicyclomine (Bentyl, Di-Spaz)
glycopyrrolate (Robinul)
L-hyoscyamine (Anaspaz, Levsin)
methscopolamine (Pamine)
oxyphencyclimine (Daricon)
propantheline (Pro-Banthine)

Drugs which combine an antispasmodic effect with the central nervous system sedative phenobarbital include:

Bellergal-S
Donnatal

The combination drug Librax contains an antispasmodic with the antianxiety agent chlordiazepoxide (Librium).

Antidiarrheal Drugs

Antidiarrheal drugs produce a therapeutic effect by slowing peristalsis in the intestinal tract or by absorbing the extra water in diarrhea stools and forming a gel. Some antidiarrheal drugs exert their effect because they contain opium or related substances. Although opium and related compounds have pain-relieving properties, a common side effect of that group of drugs is constipation. This side effect becomes a therapeutic effect in treating diarrhea.

Drugs for diarrhea which contain opium or related substances are classified as **narcotics** and may be controlled substances depending on the actual addictive qualities of that particular drug.

difenoxin (Motofen)	Schedule IV drug
diphenoxylate (Lomotil)	Schedule V drug
loperamide (Imodium)	Not a schedule drug
tincture of opium (paregoric)	Schedule III drug

Other antidiarrheal drugs contain non-opiate substances such as kaolin and pectin which absorb water. These drugs include:

Donnagel
Kaolin
Kaopectate

Laxatives

Prescription laxatives are used for short-term treatment of constipation, with attention also given to adequate water intake, dietary fiber/bulk, and other measures to promote regularity. Over-the-counter laxatives are frequently overused and even abused.

There are several classifications of laxatives. These include magnesium laxatives, irritants, bulk-producing laxatives, stool softeners, and mechanical laxatives.

Magnesium laxatives include the active ingredient of magnesium which attracts water from the bloodstream into the intestines to soften the stool. These drugs include:

>Epsom salt
>M.O.M. (milk of magnesia)
>Phillips' Milk of Magnesia

Irritant laxatives act directly on the intestinal mucosa to stimulate peristalsis. These drugs include:

>cascara
>Dulcolax
>Ex-Lax
>Feen-a-Mint
>Fletcher's Castoria
>Senokot

Bulk-producing laxatives hold water that is normally absorbed into the bloodstream from the intestines. Their laxative action is the most natural and safest of all of the laxatives. These drugs include:

>Citrucel
>Fiberall
>FiberCon
>Metamucil
>Mitrolan
>Perdiem

Laxatives which act as stool **softeners** are emulsifiers which allow water and fat in the stool to mix. These include:

>Correctol
>docusate (Colace, Surfak)

Mechanical laxatives include suppositories (such as glycerin suppositories) which directly stimulate the urge to defecate by their presence in the lower colon.

Laxatives which produce therapeutic actions other than those mentioned above include:

>Doxidan
>lactulose (Chronulac)

Bowel preps or enemas may be prescribed to evacuate the colon prior to surgical or endoscopic procedures. These include:

>Fleet enema (This is manufactured with various active ingredients.
>>Fleet is the manufacturer's name.)
>polyethylene glycol/electrolyte solution (CoLyte, Evac-Q-Kit, GoLytely, X-Prep).

Drugs for Ulcerative Colitis

The chemical compound 5-aminosalicylic acid, abbreviated as 5-ASA, is used to treat ulcerative colitis. It decreases intestinal inflammation by blocking the production of prostaglandins. The drug mesalamine (Rowasa) contains 5-ASA as the active ingredient and is administered rectally as a solution. The drug sulfasalazine (Azulfidine) is taken orally and changes into 5-ASA in the colon.

Topical corticosteroids may be prescribed to treat intestinal inflammation. These drugs are solutions or foams placed into the rectum. Examples include hydrocortisone (Cortenema, Cortifoam) and methylprednisolone (Medrol Enpak).

Gastric Stimulants

For certain disease conditions such as diabetic gastric stasis, or to facilitate emptying of the intestines prior to x-rays, or to prevent distention and paralytic ileus after major abdominal surgery, some patients are given a gastric stimulant. These drugs enhance the natural action of acetylcholine (which was described previously) by increasing peristalsis in the GI tract. These drugs include:

dexpanthenol (Ilopan)
. metoclopramide (Reglan)

Antiemetics

Antiemetic drugs are used to control nausea and vomiting which can arise from bacterial or viral illnesses of the GI tract; as a side effect of drugs, surgery, radiation, or chemotherapy; or from vertigo and motion sickness. Vomiting patients are often given antiemetics in rectal suppository form because they cannot keep the oral medications down.

Bacterial or viral illnesses may directly irritate vomiting centers in the GI tract or may, like drugs, radiation, and chemotherapy, have a systemic effect which irritates the chemoreceptor trigger zone and the vomiting center in the brain. Surgery, particularly abdominal surgery, may cause peristalsis to slow or even stop (paralytic ileus), triggering vomiting. The majority of drugs prescribed for nausea and vomiting from the above conditions act by blocking dopamine from activating receptors in the wall of the GI tract and in the chemoreceptor trigger zone and vomiting center in the brain. For severe nausea and vomiting, these drugs are prescribed.

chlorpromazine (Thorazine)
perphenazine (Trilafon)
prochlorperazine (Compazine)
triflupromazine (Vesprin)

For moderate nausea and vomiting, these drugs are prescribed.

benzquinamide (Emete-Con)
promethazine (Phenergan)
thiethylperazine (Torecan)
trimethobenzamide (Tigan)

Vertigo is caused by irritation to the inner ear (from labyrinthitis or vestibular neuritis) which upsets balance and stimulates the vomiting center. Motion sickness arises from repeated motions, such as in a car, which also overstimulate the inner ear. Drugs used to treat vertigo and motion sickness seem to act by either reducing the sensitivity of the inner ear to motion or by inhibiting the increased inner ear stimuli from reaching the chemoreceptor trigger zone and the vomiting center in the brain. Drugs used to treat vertigo and motion sickness include:

>dimenhydrinate (Dramamine)
>diphenhydramine (Benadryl)
>diphenidol (Vontrol)
>meclizine (Antivert, Bonine)
>promethazine (Phenergan)
>scopolamine (Transderm-Scōp)

Note: All of these drugs are given orally with the exception of scopolamine (Transderm-Scōp) which is manufactured as a small transdermal patch worn behind the ear.

Chemotherapy drugs are most effective against rapidly dividing cells, such as cancer cells. They also affect the rapidly dividing cells in the mucous membrane of the GI tract, causing irritation, and directly stimulate the vomiting center in the brain. The chemotherapy drugs most often associated with severe nausea and vomiting include:

>cisplatin (Platinol)
>cyclophosphamide (Cytoxan)
>dacarbazine (DTIC-Dome)
>dactinomycin (actinomycin D, Cosmegen)
>doxorubicin (Adriamycin)
>nitrogen mustard

The nausea and vomiting in response to chemotherapy can be so severe and prolonged that, without treatment, patients may elect to discontinue vital chemotherapy. Therefore, antiemetic drugs are often given prophylactically to chemotherapy patients to prevent and control nausea and vomiting. These antiemetic drugs include:

>chlorpromazine (Thorazine)
>domperidone (Motilium)—an investigational drug
>dronabinol (Marinol)
>metoclopramide (Reglan)
>nabilone (Cesamet)
>prochlorperazine (Compazine)
>trimethobenzamide (Tigan)

DID YOU KNOW? The antiemetics dronabinol (Marinol) and nabilone (Cesamet) are derived from the marijuana plant. The Latin name for the marijuana plant is *Cannabis sativa*. The active components in marijuana which produce physical and psychological effects are termed *cannabinoids*. The drug dronabinol (Marinol) is a **cannabinoid.** It is also known by its chemical name delta-9-tetrahydrocannabinol, abbreviated delta-9-THC or just THC. The other drug, nabilone (Cesamet), is a synthetic manufactured cannabinoid with a similar action.

Drugs to Dissolve Gallstones

Patients who are unable to undergo surgery to remove gallstones may be given drugs which help to dissolve those stones. The first two drugs in this category (chenodiol and ursodiol) are given orally, the last two by direct injection into the gallbladder or biliary tract.

chenodiol (Chenix)   methyl tert-butyl ether (MTBE)

ursodiol (Actigall)   monoctanoin (Moctanin)

Miscellaneous GI Drugs

cromolyn sodium (Gastrocrom)   Given orally, this drug inhibits the release of histamine and is used to treat patients with food allergies to prevent the occurrence of systemic allergic symptoms.

dehydrocholic acid (Decholin)   Used to thin bile secretions in patients prone to bile duct obstruction.

ethanolamine oleate (Ethamolin)   A **sclerosing agent** that is injected locally into esophageal varices to stop bleeding.

glutamic acid (Acidulin)   Replacement therapy for gastric acid which can be decreased in patients with pernicious anemia, allergies, and stomach cancer.

neomycin (Mycifradin)   Oral antibiotic given prophylactically before intestinal surgery to inhibit bacterial growth in intestine. It is not absorbed from the GI tract.

octreotide (Sandostatin)   Used to treat severe diarrhea caused by certain cancerous tumors of the GI tract.

omeprazole (Prilosec)   Unrelated to H_2 blockers, this drug decreases gastric acid by blocking the final step of acid production in the gastric parietal cell. Its only use at this time is for treating gastroesophageal reflux and esophagitis, not ulcers. (Note: Losec, the previous trade name for omeprazole, was changed to Prilosec to avoid confusion with Lasix.)

pancrelipase (Cotazym, Pancrease)   Replacement therapy for the digestive enzyme pancrelipase normally produced by the pancreas but deficient in patients with pancreatic disease or cancer. This drug is made from powdered pigs' pancreas.

syrup of ipecac   An over-the-counter drug used to treat poisonings, its action is to induce vomiting. This drug has been abused by patients with anorexia nervosa and bulimia who use self-induced vomiting to control their weight.

REVIEW QUESTIONS

1. What is the therapeutic action of simethicone?
2. Define the terms H_2 *receptor* and H_2 *blocker*.
3. How was the trade name Tagamet selected by the manufacturer?
4. How does the anti-ulcer drug Carafate differ in action from H_2 blockers?
5. Some drugs used to control diarrhea contain opium. True or False?
6. What is the meaning of the abbreviation M.O.M.?
7. What is unusual about the antiemetic drugs Marinol and Cesamet?

14

Musculoskeletal Drugs

Drugs prescribed to treat orthopedic conditions such as arthritis (rheumatoid and osteoarthritis), bursitis, tendinitis, gout, and muscle spasms, include aspirin, nonsteroidal anti-inflammatory drugs (NSAID), gold salts, and skeletal muscle relaxants, among others. Drugs used to relieve the minor pain of contusions, strains, and sprains are described in Chapter 26, Analgesic Drugs.

Drugs for Arthritis

The medical condition of arthritis produces symptoms of inflammation, swelling, and pain in the joints. These symptoms are due to the action of prostaglandins.

> DID YOU KNOW? Prostaglandins, which are present throughout the body and exert various effects, were so named because the first prostaglandin was originally isolated from semen from the *prost*ate *gland.*

Drugs used to treat arthritis inhibit the production of prostaglandins. These drugs include salicylic acid compounds such as aspirin, nonsteroidal anti-inflammatory drugs (NSAID), gold salts, and corticosteroids.

Salicylic acid compounds. The oldest drug used to treat arthritis is aspirin. Aspirin is also known as acetylsalicylic acid, abbreviated ASA. It has anti-inflammatory, analgesic, and antipyretic actions which make it useful in treating many diverse medical conditions. Drugs which contain aspirin or related compounds and are used to treat arthritis include:

Anacin
Arthropan
A.S.A. Enseals
Ascriptin A/D
Bayer Aspirin
Bufferin
Cama
diflunisal (Dolobid)

   Easprin
   Ecotrin
   Trilisate

Note: Because salicylic acid compounds such as aspirin are irritating to the stomach and long-term therapy with such drugs has been shown to induce ulcers, some manufacturers have taken precautions to reduce this irritation. Ecotrin is manufactured as an enteric-coated tablet which will not dissolve in stomach acid; it dissolves only to release the drug when it comes into contact with the higher pH environment of the duodenum. Ascriptin A/D, Bufferin, and Cama contain magnesium and aluminum in the tablet to act as an antacid.

  Although acetaminophen (Tylenol) is an analgesic and antipyretic like aspirin, it is seldom prescribed for rheumatoid arthritis because it is not an anti-inflammatory; it lacks the ability to inhibit the production of prostaglandins.

DID YOU KNOW? Indomethacin (Indocin) is given I.V. to premature infants who have a persistent fetal circulatory pattern with a patent ductus arteriosus. The process by which Indocin helps to close the patent ductus arteriosus and establish normal circulation is not known.

  Nonsteroidal anti-inflammatory drugs (NSAID). NSAIDs have analgesic effects and also inhibit the production of prostaglandins, but they have less of a tendency than aspirin to cause gastrointestinal side effects such as ulcers. They are similar enough to aspirin structurally that patients allergic to aspirin cannot be given NSAIDs. Nonsteroidal anti-inflammatory drugs include:

   diclofenac (Voltaren)
   fenoprofen (Nalfon)
   flurbiprofen (Ansaid)
   ibuprofen (Advil, Medipren, Nuprin) over-the-counter
    (Motrin, Rufen) prescription
   indomethacin (Indocin)
   ketoprofen (Orudis)
   ketorolac (Toradol)
   meclofenamate (Meclomen)
   naproxen (Anaprox, Naprosyn)
   piroxicam (Feldene)
   sulindac (Clinoril)
   tolmetin (Tolectin)

Note: Ketorolac (Toradol) is the only NSAID which is currently approved for I.M. administration.

  The following NSAIDs are still investigational.

   carprofen (Rimadyl)
   etodolac (Ultradol)
   isoxicam (Maxicam)

Note: The ending -*profen* is common to some generic nonsteroidal anti-inflammatory drugs.

Another arthritis drug, chemically unrelated to either aspirin or NSAIDs, is phenylbutazone (Butazolidin). This drug is used infrequently, being given only when NSAIDs are not effective.

DID YOU KNOW? Phenylbutazone (Butazolidin) is commonly used in race horses to reduce inflammation. Its slang name is *bute*. It is illegal to race a horse under treatment with phenylbutazone, and post-race urine tests look for this drug.

Gold salts. Gold salts contain actual gold (from 29% to 50% of the total drug) in capsules, or solution for injection. Gold salts are used to treat active rheumatoid arthritis. Rheumatoid arthritis is an autoimmune disease in which the patient's own macrophages attack and damage cartilage. Gold salts inhibit the activity of macrophages but cannot reverse past damage. Unlike other anti-arthritis drugs, gold salts are never prescribed for osteoarthritis as this disease is caused by degenerative wear-and-tear, not by an immune response. NSAIDs are the first line of treatment for rheumatoid arthritis, but if these fail, gold salts may be added to the treatment regimen. Gold salts include the following drugs.

> auranofin (Ridaura)
> aurothioglucose (Solganal)
> gold sodium thiomalate (Myochrysine)

Note: The chemical symbol for gold is *Au*.

An additional drug for severe rheumatoid arthritis is methotrexate (Rheumatrex). Methotrexate is a well-known chemotherapy drug. The mechanism of its therapeutic action against rheumatoid arthritis is as yet unexplained. It is prescribed only after NSAIDs and gold salts have been tried.

Corticosteroids. Corticosteroids, produced in the adrenal cortex, have a powerful anti-inflammatory action. Topical corticosteroids were discussed in Chapter 11. Corticosteroids used to treat the inflammation associated with arthritis, bursitis, and tendinitis, are given orally. Some can be injected directly into the joint (intra-articular administration). Corticosteroids include:

> betamethasone (Celestone)
> cortisone (Cortone)
> dexamethasone (Decadron)
> hydrocortisone (Cortef, Hydrocortone, Solu-Cortef)
> methylprednisolone (Depo-Medrol, Medrol, Solu-Medrol)
> prednisolone (Delta-Cortef)
> prednisone (Deltasone)
> triamcinolone (Aristocort, Aristospan, Kenacort)

For additional information on corticosteroids, see Chapter 21, page 108.

Skeletal Muscle Relaxants

Acute musculoskeletal conditions such as strains, sprains, and "pulled muscles" can be treated with analgesics and anti-inflammatory drugs; but the physician may elect to also prescribe a skeletal muscle relaxant in addition to rest and physical therapy. Skeletal muscle relaxants most specifically relieve muscle spasm and stiffness. In addition, some have a sedative quality. These drugs include:

> carisoprodol (Soma)
> chlorzoxazone (Parafon Forte DSC)
> cyclobenzaprine (Flexeril)
> diazepam (Valium)
> metaxalone (Skelaxin)
> methocarbamol (Robaxin)
> orphenadrine (Flexon, Norflex)

Combination drugs include:

> Norgesic (orphenadrine and aspirin)
> Robaxisal (methocarbamol and aspirin)
> Soma Compound (carisoprodol and aspirin)

Drugs for Gout

Gout is caused by a defect of metabolism which results in increased amounts of uric acid in the blood. This excess uric acid then crystallizes within the joints causing pain and inflammation. Drugs used to treat gout act by either increasing the excretion of uric acid in the urine or by inhibiting its production. These drugs include:

> allopurinol (Zyloprim)
> colchicine
> probenecid (Benemid)
> sulfinpyrazone (Anturane)

In addition, several nonsteroidal anti-inflammatory drugs (NSAID) discussed earlier have been found to be of particular benefit in treating gout. These include:

> indomethacin (Indocin)
> phenylbutazone (Butazolidin)
> sulindac (Clinoril)

Miscellaneous Drugs

baclofen (Lioresal)   Used to treat muscle spasticity caused by multiple sclerosis.

bupivacaine (Marcaine)   A local anesthetic injected into the joint cavity following arthroscopic surgery to relieve postoperative pain.

calcitonin (Calcimar)   A hormone normally produced by the thyroid gland which regulates calcium use by bones, this synthetic drug is used to treat postmenopausal osteoporosis.

calcitriol (Rocaltrol)   Vitamin D analog that promotes the absorption of calcium and phosphorus from the GI tract and absorption of these minerals into the bones. Used to treat osteoporosis.

chymopapain (Chymodiactin)   An enzyme which dissolves the proteins in cartilage, chymopapain is injected into a lumbar disk which has herniated and is pressing on spinal nerves. This treatment is an alternative to surgical correction.

dantrolene (Dantrium)   Used to treat muscle spasticity from spinal cord injury, stroke, cerebral palsy, or multiple sclerosis.

misoprostol (Cytotec)   Given to patients on long-term aspirin or nonsteroidal anti-inflammatory drugs (NSAID) to prevent their common side effect of gastric ulcers. Aspirin and NSAIDs inhibit the formation of prostaglandins; prostaglandins produce inflammation and pain in arthritis, but also normally act to protect the gastric mucosa. Misoprostol is a synthetic prostaglandin which protects the gastric mucosa when natural prostaglandin is inhibited by arthritis drugs.

REVIEW QUESTIONS

1. Give the meaning of these abbreviations: ASA, NSAID.
2. How does an enteric-coated aspirin tablet such as Ecotrin help prevent gastric ulcers in arthritis patients?
3. Name three over-the-counter trade names and two prescription trade names for ibuprofen.
4. Indocin is a nonsteroidal anti-inflammatory drug used to treat both arthritis and premature infants with patent ductus arteriosus. True or False?
5. Gold salts are useful in treating both osteoarthritis and rheumatoid arthritis. True or False?

SPELLING TIPS

- Several gold salts drugs contain *au,* the chemical symbol for gold: **au**ranofin, Rid**au**ra, **au**rothioglucose.
- Flexeril (Often misspelled as *Flexoril* because of association with the flexor muscle.)

15

Cardiovascular Drugs

Cardiovascular drugs are used to treat a variety of conditions, including congestive heart failure, angina pectoris, arrhythmias, hypertension, hypertensive crisis, and hyperlipidemia.

Drugs for Congestive Heart Failure

Congestive heart failure occurs when the heart muscle is weakened and unable to adequately pump blood. Right-sided heart failure results in a backup of blood in the venous circulation, producing liver enlargement and edema in the extremities. Left-sided heart failure results in a backup of blood in the pulmonary circulation producing pulmonary edema.

The **cardiac glycosides** are a group of chemically related drugs, prescribed for congestive heart failure, whose molecular structure consists of chains of glucose sugars known as glycosides; hence the name *cardiac glycosides.*

In ancient times, cardiac glycosides were extracted from the dried foxglove plant (Latin name, *Digitalis*). Today, these drugs are extracted and purified or synthetically produced. The term *digitalis* refers collectively to all of the cardiac glycosides.

Cardiac glycosides are used to treat congestive heart failure; this application is based on the two separate medical effects of cardiac glycosides which allow the heart to pump more slowly but more efficiently.

• **Positive inotropic effect.** This refers to the ability of the cardiac glycosides to increase the strength of cardiac contractions. They do so by inhibiting the flow of positive sodium ions into the cell, allowing more positive calcium ions to enter. This increased level of intracellular calcium results in a stronger contraction of cells of the myocardium. Note: *Ino-* refers to *(cardiac muscle) fibers.*

• **Negative chronotropic effect.** This refers to the ability of the cardiac glycosides to slow the heart rate. This is accomplished by the release of acetylcholine which depresses the SA node and slows electrical conduction. In combination with the positive inotropic effect, this negative chronotropic effect allows the heart to pump more efficiently and fill completely before the next contraction--an important therapeutic action for patients with congestive heart failure. The negative chronotropic effect is also the therapeutic effect used to treat atrial flutter/fibrillation as discussed later in this chapter. Note: *Chrono-* refers to the *time* of a heartbeat.

HISTORICAL NOTE: In the 1500s foxglove was given the botanical name *Digitalis* which referred to its fingerlike flowers (like the digits of the hand). In the 1780s, an English physician published a book on foxglove and its medical uses. He stated, "My opinion was asked concerning a family recipe for the cure of dropsy [an old term for the symptoms of congestive heart failure]. I was told that it had long been kept a secret by an old woman in Shropshire who had sometimes made cures after the more regular practitioners had failed. I was informed also that the effects produced were violent vomiting. . . . This medicine was composed of twenty or more different herbs; but it was not very difficult for one conversant in these subjects to perceive that the active herb could be no other than foxglove."

Michael C. Gerald, *Pharmacology: An Introduction to Drugs,* 2nd ed. (Englewood Cliffs, N.J.: Prentice-Hall, Inc., 1981), p. 402

The cardiac glycosides used to treat congestive heart failure include:

deslanoside (Cedilanid-D)

digitoxin (Crystodigin)

digoxin (Lanoxin, Lanoxicaps)

Note: Digoxin is by far the most commonly prescribed cardiac glycoside. This is because it has a **shorter half-life** than the other cardiac glycosides and therefore less chance of causing toxicity. Deslanoside is only administered I.M. or I.V.

Digitalis toxicity from cardiac glycosides is a serious and frequent adverse effect. Nearly one-third of patients taking a cardiac glycoside develop symptoms of digitalis toxicity. This is because these drugs have a low therapeutic index (i.e., there is a narrow margin between the therapeutic dose and the toxic dose), and **long half-life** which is even more prolonged in elderly patients with decreased kidney function. Symptoms of toxicity may include a pulse rate below 60 beats per minute, confusion, fatigue, nausea/vomiting, diarrhea, or yellow-green halos around lights.

To prevent toxic effects, physicians order blood tests to determine the level of digitalis in the blood. These are often referred to as "dig levels" (pronounced "dij"). Symptoms from toxicity may be treated by changing the dosage to a less frequent schedule or, in severe cases, by administering digoxin immune fab (Digibind). For a description of this drug, see Miscellaneous Drugs at the end of the chapter.

Other drugs for congestive heart failure. Diuretics are often combined with cardiac glycosides to treat patients with congestive heart failure. Diuretics act to increase the excretion of sodium and water to reduce edema, a common symptom of congestive heart failure. For a complete discussion of diuretics, see Chapter 12.

There are other drugs for congestive heart failure which increase the strength of contraction of the heart muscle but which do not belong to the cardiac glycoside class of drugs. These other drugs are only prescribed for patients who have not responded to cardiac glycosides and diuretics. They include:

amrinone (Inocor)

milrinone (Primacor)—an investigational drug

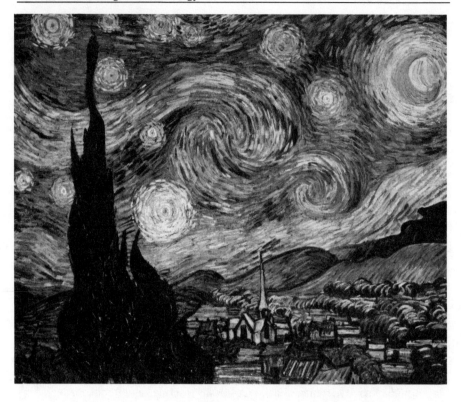

FIGURE 15-1

Digitalis toxicity. Vincent van Gogh's "The Starry Night" (1889) is felt by some physicians to show evidence of digitalis toxicity in the way the Dutch painter depicted yellow-green halos around the stars. Van Gogh (1853-1890) suffered from mania and epilepsy and may have been given digitalis for lack of a more specific drug therapy available at that time. Photo, oil on canvas, 29 x 36¼'', Collection, The Museum of Modern Art, New York. Acquired through the Lillie P. Bliss Bequest. Reprinted with permission.

Antianginal Drugs

The pain of angina pectoris occurs when cells of the myocardium receive insufficiently oxygenated blood to meet their needs. This can occur due to an increased need for oxygen during exercise, stress, due to increased **afterload** (the pressure of the arterial system against which the heart must pump), or increased **preload** (the pressure of the venous system supplying the heart with blood). Angina can also occur because of decreased oxygen supply due to plaques in the coronary arteries, spasm of the coronary arteries, or from the vasoconstrictive effect of smoking. The pain of angina pectoris denotes cellular ischemia but not cellular death. If untreated, however, this ischemia can progress to cellular death, i.e., a myocardial infarction.

The drugs used to treat angina include nitrates, beta blockers, and calcium channel blockers, as discussed below.

Nitrates used to treat angina. As a group, nitrates act as vasodilators throughout the vascular system. By dilating veins, they reduce preload and decrease the need of the myocardium for oxygen. They also increase the flow of oxygenated blood through the coronary arteries.

The most frequently prescribed nitrate is nitroglycerin. All of the nitrates, including nitroglycerin, can be administered in several different ways:

> sublingually as a spray
> sublingually as a tablet
> transmucosally between the cheek and gum as a tablet
> orally as a sustained-release capsule
> transdermally as a patch
> topically as an ointment (measured in inches)
> intravenously

However, not every nitrate can be administered by every route.

The trade names for nitroglycerin include:

> Minitran
> Nitro-Bid
> Nitrocap T.D.
> Nitrodisc
> Nitro-Dur
> Nitrogard
> Nitrol
> Nitrolingual
> Nitrong
> Nitrospan
> Nitrostat
> Transderm-Nitro
> Tridil

Other nitrates include:

> erythrityl tetranitrate (Cardilate)
> isosorbide dinitrate (Isordil, Sorbitrate)
> pentaerythritol tetranitrate (Peritrate, P.E.T.N.)

Beta blockers used to treat angina. Although nitrates, particularly nitroglycerin, comprise the standard for antianginal therapy, beta blockers may also be prescribed. Beta blockers act to decrease the heart rate which in turn decreases the need of the myocardium for oxygen; this decreases anginal pain. (A more detailed description of beta-blocker therapeutic action and beta receptors is provided later in this chapter.)

Beta blockers used to treat angina include:

> atenolol (Tenormin)
> metoprolol (Lopressor)
> nadolol (Corgard)
> propranolol (Inderal)

Note: The ending -olol is common to generic beta blockers.

For patients who have had a myocardial infarction, the beta blockers propranolol (Inderal) and timolol (Blocadren) are prescribed to reduce the risk of a second heart attack.

Not all beta blockers are indicated for treating angina. Beta blockers are also used to treat hypertension and arrhythmias. These applications are discussed later in this chapter.

Calcium channel blockers used to treat angina. Calcium channel blockers may be used in conjunction with nitrates or beta blockers to treat angina. Calcium channel blockers relax the smooth muscle of the blood vessels to decrease arterial pressure, the pressure the heart must pump against. This decreases the heart's need for oxygen. This same action also dilates the coronary arteries and prevents coronary artery spasm which can trigger angina.

IN DEPTH: On a cellular level, calcium channel blockers act in the following way. The pumping contraction of the heart muscle as well as the contraction of smooth muscle of blood vessels depends on the flow of calcium ions from outside to inside each cell. These calcium ions move into the cell in a specific way, through what have been termed calcium channels. Calcium channel blockers prevent the movement of calcium from outside the cell through these channels to inside the cell. With less calcium inside the cell, it contracts less strongly and less often. This effect at a cellular level is demonstrated throughout the body as the smooth muscle around the blood vessels relaxes, and the heart contracts less forcefully and less frequently.

Calcium channel blockers used to treat angina include:
diltiazem (Cardizem)
nicardipine (Cardene)
nifedipine (Adalat, Procardia)
verapamil (Calan, Isoptin, Verelan)
Note: The ending *-ipine* is common to some generic calcium channel blocking drugs.

Aspirin. One tablet of aspirin daily has been shown to significantly decrease the incidence of a second heart attack because of its anticoagulant effect.

Antiarrhythmic Drugs

Cardiac arrhythmias are caused by abnormalities in the normal conduction of electrical impulses from the SA node through the AV node, bundle of His, and Purkinje system in the heart. Disruptions in this conduction pattern and changes in the normal period of time between beats (the refractory period) result in various arrhythmias involving the atria or ventricles. Arrhythmias can manifest as bradycardia, tachycardia, atrial flutter (very rapid contraction of the atria not coordinated with the ventricle), ventricular fibrillation (ineffective, extremely rapid contractions of the ventricle), or irregularly spaced beats (bigeminy, premature contractions, heart block).

Most antiarrhythmic drugs exert a therapeutic effect by acting at different times in various ways during the electrical cycle of the heart. Some antiarrhythmic drugs exert their effect during depolarization of myocardial cells; other antiarrhythmic drugs exert their effect during repolarization, when the cell returns to its original resting state. But the action of each is based on the slowing of the rapid flow of positive sodium ions from outside to inside the cell.

Note: The EKG provides a visual representation of this cycle of events. Depolarization of the atria and ventricles corresponds to the P and QRS waves respectively; repolarization of the ventricles corresponds to the T wave.

In addition to the standard antiarrhythmic drugs described above, beta blockers are also prescribed for ventricular arrhythmias. They act by blocking beta receptors in the heart from responding to epinephrine. Epinephrine is normally released by the sympathetic nervous system and acts to increase the heart rate. By blocking the effects of epinephrine at beta receptors in the heart, beta blockers are effective in slowing the heart rate and controlling arrhythmias.

Antiarrhythmic drugs used to treat both atrial and ventricular arrhythmias include:
 acecainide (Napa)—an investigational drug
 cifenline succinate (Cipralan)—an investigational drug
 procainamide (Procan SR, Pronestyl)
 propranolol (Inderal)—a beta blocker drug
 quinidine (Cardioquin, Duraquin, Quinaglute, Quinidex)
Antiarrhythmic drugs indicated only for ventricular arrhythmias include:
 adenosine (Adenocard)
 bretylium tosylate (Bretylol)
 disopyramide (Norpace)
 lidocaine (Xylocaine)
 mexiletine (Mexitil)
 tocainide (Tonocard)

 acebutolol (Sectral)—a beta blocker
 atenolol (Tenormin)—a beta blocker
 esmolol (Brevibloc)—a beta blocker
 metoprolol (Lopressor)—a beta blocker
 nadolol (Corgard)—a beta blocker
 pindolol (Visken)—a beta blocker
 propranolol (Inderal)—a beta blocker
 timolol (Blocadren)—a beta blocker
 verapamil (Calan, Isoptin)—a calcium channel blocker
Antiarrhythmic drugs indicated only for life-threatening arrhythmias or those arrhythmias which do not respond to the previously mentioned drugs include:
 amiodarone (Cordarone)
 encainide (Enkaid)
 flecainide (Tambocor)

indecainide (Decabid)—an investigational drug
moricizine (Ethmozine)
propafenone (Rythmol)

Other drugs used to treat arrhythmias. The **cardiac glycosides** (digoxin, digitoxin) also have an antiarrhythmic effect in that they slow the heart rate. This is accomplished by the release of acetylcholine which depresses the SA node and slows electrical conduction. This therapeutic effect is used to treat atrial flutter/fibrillation.

The antiarrhythmic drug atropine is used to treat bradycardia, but its action differs from that of most antiarrhythmic drugs. It blocks the action of acetylcholine which is normally released by the parasympathetic nervous system to slow the heart rate. With the action of acetylcholine blocked, the too-slow heart rate increases.

DID YOU KNOW? The antiarrhythmic drug lidocaine (Xylocaine) is also a popular local anesthetic. Its action locally is similar to its antiarrhythmic action: it inhibits the flow of sodium into the cell. In the heart, this slows the electrical impulse that would cause the heart to contract. As an anesthetic, lidocaine inhibits sodium as well and, because the drug is much more concentrated locally, it actually stops electrical impulses along sensory nerves. With no impulses traveling along sensory nerves, there is no transmission/perception of pain.

Antihypertensive Drugs

Hypertension is a condition which manifests itself as an increase in systolic and/or diastolic blood pressure. Hypertension is caused by arteriosclerosis or kidney disease, or other diseases, or it may have no identified cause; this last type is known as essential hypertension.

Several classes of drugs are used to treat hypertension. These include diuretics, beta blockers, calcium channel blockers, ACE inhibitors, alpha receptor blockers, and vasodilators. In addition, most patients are asked to restrict the use of salt in cooking and at the table, or the physician may prescribe a low-salt diet which places a limit on total dietary sodium intake.

The treatment of hypertension follows what is known as a **step-care approach.** One antihypertensive agent, often a diuretic, is prescribed first. If a satisfactory reduction in blood pressure is not achieved, a second antihypertensive agent, such as a beta blocker, is added. Beta blockers may also be selected as the first step of treatment. Other drugs, as mentioned above, are added to the treatment regimen as necessary to achieve control of blood pressure.

Diuretics used to treat hypertension. By promoting the excretion of sodium and water, diuretics decrease total blood volume and blood pressure. For a complete discussion of this class of drugs, see Chapter 12, page 57.

Beta blockers used to treat hypertension. Beta blockers are used to treat hypertension because they cause the heart to beat less frequently and they also dilate the blood vessels; these actions contribute to a lower blood pressure.

IN DEPTH: Beta receptors are special protein molecules located in the cells of the heart and in the smooth muscle of blood vessels and bronchi. Those in the heart are designated beta$_1$ or ß$_1$ receptors. Those in the smooth muscle of blood vessels or bronchi are designated beta$_2$ or ß$_2$ receptors. Beta receptors are normally stimulated by epinephrine released by the sympathetic nervous system. When **beta$_1$ receptors** in the heart are stimulated, they cause the heart rate to increase. When **beta$_2$ receptors** in smooth muscle are stimulated, they cause the blood vessels to constrict. These two responses result in a rise in blood pressure. In addition, when beta$_2$ receptors in the smooth muscle of the bronchi are stimulated, they cause the bronchi to relax, increasing air flow to the lungs.

All of these effects are desirable because it is the job of the sympathetic nervous system to raise the blood pressure and take in more oxygen to prepare the body for fight or flight. However, in patients with hypertension or angina, these effects are not desirable. Therefore hypertensive patients are given a drug which can block the action of epinephrine on beta receptors; these drugs are termed beta blockers.

Drugs which block both beta$_1$ and beta$_2$ receptors are termed **nonselective beta blockers.** Other drugs have been developed to be more selective and block only beta$_1$ receptors in the heart; these drugs are termed **cardioselective beta blockers.**

Hypertensive patients with asthma would not be prescribed nonselective beta blockers because the beta$_2$ blocking action in the bronchi would cause bronchial constriction. Cardioselective beta blockers which have no effect on the bronchi are the treatment of choice for these patients.

Nonselective beta blockers used to treat hypertension include:
> carteolol (Cartrol)
> dilevalol (Unicard)—an investigational drug
> labetalol (Normodyne, Trandate)
> nadolol (Corgard)
> penbutolol (Levatol)
> pindolol (Visken)
> propranolol (Inderal)
> timolol (Blocadren)

Cardioselective beta blockers used to treat hypertension include:
> acebutolol (Sectral)
> atenolol (Tenormin)

betaxolol (Kerlone)
esmolol (Brevibloc)
metoprolol (Lopressor)
Note: The ending *-olol* is common to many generic beta blocking drugs.

DID YOU KNOW? Propranolol (Inderal) is used to prevent migraine headaches. Its mechanism of action is unknown.

Calcium channel blockers used to treat hypertension. Some calcium channel blockers are used to treat hypertension. They exert a therapeutic effect by relaxing the smooth muscle of blood vessels and causing them to dilate, thereby decreasing blood pressure.

Calcium channel blockers used to treat hypertension include:
diltiazem (Cardizem)
isradipine (DynaCirc)—an investigational drug
nicardipine (Cardene)
nifedipine (Adalat, Procardia)
nitrendipine (Baypress)—an investigational drug
verapamil (Calan, Isoptin, Verelan)

ACE inhibitors used to treat hypertension. Angiotensin converting enzyme (ACE) inhibitors have an antihypertensive action that is distinctly different from that of other drugs described previously. They act by both dilating arterial blood vessels and by decreasing blood volume in the following way.

IN DEPTH: The body has its own natural blood pressure-regulating system. In response to low blood pressure, the kidneys secrete renin which then helps to synthesize angiotensin I. Angiotensin I is a relatively inactive substance until, when acted upon by angiotensin converting enzyme (ACE), it becomes angiotensin II, a strong vasoconstrictor. Angiotensin II not only constricts blood vessels to raise the blood pressure, but it also stimulates the adrenal glands to produce aldosterone. Aldosterone inhibits the excretion of sodium and water from the kidneys which increases blood volume and raises the blood pressure. ACE inhibitors, when used to treat hypertension, act by breaking this cycle. ACE inhibitors prevent angiotensin converting enzyme from changing angiotensin I into angiotensin II. Because of this action, the blood vessels dilate and less aldosterone is produced so that the blood volume decreases. These two effects lower the blood pressure.

ACE inhibitors used to treat hypertension include:
captopril (Capoten)
enalapril (Vasotec)

lisinopril (Prinivil, Zestril)

Note: The ending *-pril* is common to generic ACE inhibitors.

Drugs Used to Treat Hypertensive Crisis

A patient in hypertensive crisis exhibits an extremely high blood pressure; this is a life-threatening emergency. Drugs given to treat this condition include:

    diazoxide (Hyperstat)

    nifedipine (Adalat, Procardia)

    nitroprusside (Nipride)

Note: Nitroprusside and diazoxide are given I.V., while nifedipine is given orally; the capsule is punctured and the contents placed sublingually for an immediate anti-hypertensive effect.

Antiadrenergic drugs used to treat hypertension. Adrenergic receptors of the sympathetic nervous system consist of both alpha and beta receptors, although anti-adrenergic drugs as a designated class of drugs act only to block alpha receptors. Antiadrenergic drugs which act centrally to block alpha receptors in the brain do so by blocking the natural neurotransmitter norepinephrine. As a feedback mechanism, less norepinephrine is produced and blood vessels dilate.

Centrally acting antiadrenergic drugs used to treat hypertension include:

    clonidine (Catapres)

    guanabenz (Wytensin)

    guanfacine (Tenex)

    methyldopa (Aldomet)

DID YOU KNOW? Clonidine has also been used to relieve the symptoms of nicotine withdrawal in patients who have quit smoking.

Some antiadrenergic drugs act directly at the site of blood vessels by blocking the action of norepinephrine at receptors on the blood vessels. This causes the blood vessels to dilate.

Peripherally acting antiadrenergic drugs used to treat hypertension include:

    deserpidine (Harmonyl)

    guanadrel (Hylorel)

    guanethidine (Ismelin)

    rescinnamine (Moderil)

    reserpine (Serpasil)

More specific antiadrenergic drugs have been developed which have been given a special designation as $alpha_1$ adrenergic blockers.

$Alpha_1$ adrenergic blockers used to treat hypertension include:

    doxazosin mesylate (Cardura)—an investigational drug

    prazosin (Minipress)

    terazosin (Hytrin)

Note: The ending *-azosin* is common to generic $alpha_1$ blocking drugs.

Vasodilators used to treat hypertension. Vasodilator drugs block the movement of calcium into the smooth muscle around the blood vessels. The less calcium in the smooth muscle cell, the less strongly it contracts. By relaxing smooth muscle, the blood vessel dilates and the blood pressure decreases.

Note: Although calcium channel blockers act in a similar way to vasodilators, they remain two separate classifications of antihypertensives which are not structurally related to each other.

Vasodilators used to treat hypertension include:

hydralazine (Apresoline)
minoxidil (Loniten, Minodyl)
pinacidil (Pindac)—an investigational drug

DID YOU KNOW? Minoxidil is also marketed under the trade name Rogaine and is used to treat male pattern baldness. Applied topically, its vasodilator action reestablishes blood flow to hair follicles, resulting in new hair growth in some patients.

Antihypertensive/Diuretic Drugs

The following drugs combine an antihypertensive agent with a diuretic:

Aldoril (methyldopa and hydrochlorothiazide)
Apresazide (hydralazine and hydrochlorothiazide)
Capozide (captopril and hydrochlorothiazide)
Combipres (clonidine and chlorthalidone)
Diupres (reserpine and chlorothiazide)
Enduronyl (deserpidine and methyclothiazide)
Hydromox R (reserpine and quinethazone)
Inderide (propranolol and hydrochlorothiazide)
Minizide (prazosin and polythiazide)
Renese-R (reserpine and polythiazide)
Ser-Ap-Es (reserpine, hydralazine, and hydrochlorothiazide)
Tenoretic (atenolol and chlorthalidone)
Timolide (timolol and hydrochlorothiazide)
Vaseretic (enalapril and hydrochlorothiazide)
Zestoretic (lisinopril and hydrochlorothiazide)

Peripheral Vasodilators

Peripheral vasodilators are used not to treat hypertension but to increase peripheral blood flow to treat diseases such as arteriosclerosis obliterans, Buerger disease, Raynaud disease, and diabetic peripheral vascular insufficiency. These drugs act selectively to dilate arteries in skeletal muscles:

isoxsuprine (Vasodilan)
nylidrin (Arlidin)

Hyperlipidemia Drugs

Hyperlipidemia is a general term encompassing both hypercholesterolemia (increased levels of serum cholesterol) and hypertriglyceridemia (increased levels of serum triglycerides). Hyperlipidemia is one of several well-defined risk factors for atherosclerosis; others include smoking, obesity, hypertension, stress, and sedentary life-style.

Cholesterol is normally produced by the liver. A certain amount of cholesterol is needed by the body for the production of hormones and as a normal component of skin and nerve fibers. Excess dietary cholesterol, however, can cause elevated serum levels. Dietary sources of cholesterol include foods of animal origin, such as fatty meat, egg yolks, bacon, shrimp, cream, lard, etc. Some patients develop extremely high cholesterol levels unrelated to dietary intake of cholesterol because they have a genetic disorder in which there are insufficient receptors for cholesterol to bind to.

Triglycerides are normally produced by the liver. Certain amounts of triglycerides are used to produce subcutaneous fat which cushions and protects the body. Excess dietary levels of nonanimal fats can result in larger than normal storage of fat in the body. It is also of interest to note that excess dietary sugar is converted into triglycerides and stored as body fat. Dietary sources of triglycerides include oils, margarine, and sugar.

DID YOU KNOW? Alcoholics often have extremely elevated serum triglyceride levels. The excess calories consumed in drinking alcoholic beverages are converted to triglycerides.

Just as water and oil do not mix, so fats or lipids (cholesterol and triglycerides) do not mix in the serum. Therefore, in order to be transported through the blood, cholesterol and triglycerides must bind to certain proteins. The combination of these lipids and proteins is known as lipoproteins. There are three classes of lipoproteins found in the body. They are:

HDL (high-density lipoproteins)
LDL (low-density lipoproteins)
VLDL (very low-density lipoproteins)

The functions of these lipoproteins are quite different. HDL removes excess serum cholesterol, carrying it away from cells to the liver where it is excreted in the bile; therefore, high levels of HDL are desirable. LDL carries excess cholesterol from the serum to receptors on a cell membrane where it is metabolized for energy or deposited on artery walls to form arteriosclerotic plaques; thus, high levels of LDL are undesirable. VLDL carries triglycerides, and so high levels of VLDL are undesirable.

Antihyperlipidemia drugs act to either increase levels of HDL, decrease levels of LDL, or decrease levels of VLDL.

Dietary therapy rather than drug therapy is the first choice of treatment for hyperlipidemia. In addition, exercise and weight loss may be recommended. Decreased alcohol intake may also be recommended.

Drugs which reduce serum cholesterol levels act by causing more cholesterol to be excreted in the bile or by decreasing levels of LDL. The first two drugs are known specifically as **bile acid sequestrants**, while the other drugs are simply antihyperlipemic agents.

> cholestyramine (Cholybar, Questran)
> colestipol (Colestid)
> dextrothyroxine (Choloxin)
> lovastatin (Mevacor)
> probucol (Lorelco)

Drugs which reduce serum triglyceride levels act by decreasing the levels of VLDL. These drugs include:

> clofibrate (Atromid-S)
> gemfibrozil (Lopid)

Some nonprescription dietary supplements which are used to lower VLDL and LDL levels and raise HDL levels to treat both hypercholesterolemia and hypertriglyceridemia include:

> niacin (nicotinic acid, Nicolar)
> omega-3 fatty acids (Promega, Proto-Chol)

Emergency Cardiac Drugs

Emergency drugs used in cardiovascular resuscitation are discussed in Chapter 16, page 88.

Anticoagulant/Thrombolytic Drugs

Anticoagulant and thrombolytic drugs are discussed in Chapter 17, page 92.

Miscellaneous Drugs

alprostadil (prostaglandin E_1, Prostin VR) A prostaglandin drug which produces vasodilation and relaxation of smooth muscle. Vasodilation improves blood flow and oxygenation while keeping the smooth muscle of the ductus arteriosus open. This is therapeutic in newborn infants with congenital heart defects who need to have the ductus arteriosus remain patent to provide oxygenated blood to the body until surgical correction can be accomplished and anatomically correct circulation restored.

digoxin immune fab (Digibind) Administered I.V. to treat life-threatening digitalis toxicity, this drug is obtained from sheep which have been treated to produce antibodies against the basic molecule common to all the cardiac glycosides.

dipyridamole (Persantine) A coronary artery dilator, this drug is no longer indicated for angina but is used during thallium testing for patients with coronary artery disease who cannot tolerate an exercise stress test. Normally, exercise on a treadmill is used to induce angina in these patients. Since they cannot exercise, dipyridamole is given to dilate the arteries, causing the heart rate to reflexly increase. This will provoke angina in these patients and result in a positive test.

Fluosol A solution of water and chemicals which can dissolve oxygen and carbon dioxide, Fluosol is injected directly into the coronary arteries to prevent ischemic changes and damage to the myocardium during PTCA or balloon angioplasty procedures.

indomethacin (Indocin) Given I.V., this drug is used to close a patent ductus arteriosus in premature infants with persistent fetal circulation. The mechanism by which it exerts its action is not known.

penicillin G Used prophylactically to prevent bacterial endocarditis in patients with congenital heart disease or rheumatic heart disease undergoing dental procedures and other surgery.

pentoxifylline (Trental) Unrelated to either peripheral vasodilators or anticoagulants, this drug acts to decrease blood viscosity to improve blood flow through peripheral and cerebral arteries.

tolazoline (Priscoline) Used to decrease pulmonary hypertension in newborns with persistent fetal circulation who cannot maintain adequate levels of oxygenation. Given I.V. only.

vitamin B$_{12}$ (cyanocobalamin) Necessary for red blood cell formation, absorption of vitamin B$_{12}$ depends on the presence of intrinsic factor in the stomach. Intrinsic factor is decreased in pernicious anemia, and B$_{12}$ is usually given by I.M. injection, although, in high enough doses, B$_{12}$ can be given orally if oral intrinsic factor is also given (as combined in the drug Trinsicon).

REVIEW QUESTIONS

1. What two basic therapeutic effects do cardiac glycosides have on the heart?
2. Name the most commonly prescribed cardiac glycoside drug for congestive heart failure.
3. As a student of both pharmacology and art history, what insightful, thoughtful comment might you make concerning Vincent van Gogh's painting, "The Starry Night"?
4. The ending *-olol* is common to generic calcium channel blockers. True or False?
5. Beta blockers can be used to treat angina, hypertension, and arrhythmias. True or False?
6. Name five routes by which nitroglycerin can be administered.
7. Sheep's antibodies : Digibind = foxglove : _____.
   A. *Digitalis* plant
   B. Lanoxin
   C. DynaCirc
   D. Cardioquin
8. What does the *SR* in Procan SR indicate? (Clue: See also under "SR" on page 43.)
9. What antiarrhythmic drug is also a popular local anesthetic?
10. What do the drugs Mevacor, Lorelco, and Questran have in common?

16

Emergency Drugs

When a patient's cardiac or respiratory function decreases, a life-threatening condition exists. This decrease in function may be due to a variety of causes such as myocardial infarction, ventricular fibrillation, respiratory failure, or drug overdose. When a patient experiences cardiac and respiratory arrest, there is a cessation of spontaneous respirations with either absence of the heart beat (asystole) or the presence of such severe arrhythmias as to negate cardiac output. Unless these life-threatening problems can be corrected within a matter of minutes, carbon dioxide (pCO_2) and lactic acid levels in the blood will rise rapidly, the blood pH will become more acidic, and cell metabolism in the vital organs will slowly come to a halt; the patient will die.

Basic life support measures as performed in cardiopulmonary resuscitation (CPR) involve mechanically circulating the blood and inflating the lungs. Advanced cardiac life support (ACLS) also includes the use of drug therapy. The type of emergency drug selected is based on the patient's symptoms. Drugs are used to maintain heart rate and blood pressure and to correct serum pH imbalances. Intravenous lines are inserted to provide access for drug administration. A **crash cart** containing all necessary emergency drugs and resuscitative equipment (including defibrillator paddles) is available in every patient area in the hospital.

The following routes of administration are used for emergency drugs.

intravenous Drugs are given by intravenous push or **bolus** to produce a maximum drug effect in the shortest period of time. Following successful resuscitation, continuous I.V. drip infusion is then used. The intravenous route is by far the most common way of administering emergency drugs.

endotracheal An alternative route to intravenous is endotracheal. Drugs are administered by injecting the solution into the endotracheal tube that is used to ventilate the patient. As the lungs are mechanically ventilated, the drug solution is rapidly absorbed by the lung tissue into the pulmonary capillary network. Therapeutic serum drug levels can be attained that equal those of intravenous administration; however, only certain drugs can be administered endotracheally. These drugs include epinephrine (Adrenalin), atropine, lidocaine (Xylocaine), and naloxone (Narcan). Note: Narcan is a narcotic antagonist given only to patients with suspected narcotic overdose.

intracardiac This route is not frequently used but can be valuable when other routes have failed to produce a therapeutic result. This route carries with it the risk of pneumothorax, cardiac tamponade, or coronary artery laceration if the injection is not properly placed into the left ventricular chamber. Only epinephrine (Adrenalin) and atropine are given by this route.

For emergency purposes, all other routes of administration result in too slow an absorption rate for the drug to produce therapeutic results before the patient dies.

Drugs commonly given during emergency resuscitation include epinephrine (Adrenalin), lidocaine (Xylocaine), atropine, sodium bicarbonate, calcium chloride, and vasopressors.

Epinephrine. Epinephrine (Adrenalin) normally is produced in the body and released by the action of the sympathetic nervous system. The body's physiologic response to epinephrine involves:

- Constriction of blood vessels due to stimulation of alpha receptors. This raises the blood pressure.
- Increased heart rate and cardiac output due to stimulation of $beta_1$ receptors in the heart muscle.
- Relaxation of bronchial smooth muscle resulting in bronchodilation, due to stimulation of $beta_2$ receptors. Note: The latter action is of particular significance in the treatment of serious asthma attacks and will be discussed in Chapter 18.

During a cardiac arrest, epinephrine (Adrenalin) is used to increase the rate and force with which the heart beats. It is not useful for correcting cardiac arrhythmias. However, if the heart is in ventricular fibrillation, epinephrine (Adrenalin) makes the myocardium more responsive to the use of a defibrillator to restore normal rhythm. If the heart has completely stopped beating (asystole), epinephrine (Adrenalin) can actually stimulate contractions of the myocardium. It also constricts the blood vessels and raises the blood pressure. Thus, while epinephrine (Adrenalin) stimulates the heart to beat, it also helps to maintain perfusion to the heart and brain to improve the chances for a successful resuscitative effort.

Lidocaine. Lidocaine (Xylocaine) is indicated for the management of life-threatening ventricular fibrillation, and is the drug of choice in resuscitative efforts for patients with this problem. It has no therapeutic effect if the heart is in asystole.

A description of lidocaine's therapeutic action is given in Chapter 15, where other drugs for life-threatening ventricular arrhythmias are also described.

Atropine. Atropine blocks the action of acetylcholine released from the vagus nerve. The vagus nerve is part of the parasympathetic nervous system with branches that innervate the myocardium at the SA and AV nodes. When acetylcholine is released, the heart rate slows. Atropine blocks that action and is used specifically to treat bradycardia.

Sodium bicarbonate. During cardiac and respiratory arrest, the blood pH decreases rapidly as waste products accumulate in the blood. In this environment of severe acidosis, all types of emergency drug therapy lose their effectiveness. Sodium bicarbonate corrects the acidosis and returns the blood pH to within normal range. There is some controversy, however, as to the true effectiveness of sodium bicarbonate. Some studies suggest it may actually increase acidosis through a chemical reaction which releases more CO_2 into the blood.

DID YOU KNOW? Sodium bicarbonate is given orally as an antacid to neutralize excess acid in the stomach. It is marketed under the trade names Alka-Seltzer and Bromo Seltzer, and is also the active ingredient in home remedies for indigestion that contain baking soda.

Calcium chloride. Calcium chloride can stimulate the myocardium to contract more forcefully and may even stimulate a contraction when the heart is in asystole and has failed to respond to epinephrine.

Vasopressors

Drugs in this class are used to increase blood pressure, and treatment with them is begun after the patient has been resuscitated. They are given by I.V. drip. All of these drugs stimulate $beta_1$ receptors to increase the heart rate; they also stimulate alpha receptors in the blood vessels to produce vasoconstriction and raise the blood pressure. This class of drugs includes:

> dobutamine (Dobutrex)
> dopamine (Intropin)
> isoproterenol (Isuprel)
> norepinephrine (Levophed)

Vasopressors also have the desirable effect of maintaining blood flow to the kidneys so that kidney ischemia from hypotension does not later result in renal failure which would complicate an otherwise successful resuscitative effort.

DID YOU KNOW? Injectable epinephrine (Adrenalin) is included in insect bite kits. Those individuals with a life-threatening allergic reaction (anaphylaxis) when bitten can inject a premeasured dose of epinephrine subcutaneously.

Any allergic reaction involves the release of histamine. In anaphylaxis, massive amounts of histamine are released, resulting in extensive generalized vasodilation. If untreated, this causes a drop in blood pressure severe enough to produce shock. Histamine is also a powerful bronchoconstrictor. The massive amounts of histamine released during anaphylaxis can actually decrease the air movement in and out of the lungs so completely that the patient suffocates unless treatment occurs within minutes to obtain bronchodilation. Subcutaneous epinephrine given immediately after the insect bite reverses both of the above actions of histamine by constricting blood vessels to maintain a normal blood pressure and by relaxing bronchial smooth muscle to allow adequate air flow.

REVIEW QUESTIONS

1. Name the drug of choice for resuscitating patients with ventricular arrhythmias.
2. List four emergency drugs that can be given via an endotracheal tube.
3. What are the hazards of administering emergency drugs via the intracardiac route?
4. What emergency drug is given to counteract bradycardia?
5. State the arguments for and against using sodium bicarbonate intravenously during a resuscitation attempt.

17

Anticoagulants and Thrombolytic Enzymes

Anticoagulants

Blood coagulates to form a clot following a complex series of steps involving clotting factors I through XIII and platelets. Anticoagulants act to stop this process by inhibiting one or several clotting factors.

Anticoagulant drugs include:

anisindione (Miradon)
dicumarol
heparin (Calciparine)
warfarin (Coumadin)

All of these drugs are given orally with the exception of heparin which is given only subcutaneously or I.V. Hospitalized patients receiving heparin are switched to an oral anticoagulant on discharge to home. Heparin doses are measured in units.

Other anticoagulant drugs include platelet antiaggregant drugs which act by inhibiting platelets from clumping, an integral part of the clotting process. These drugs include:

aspirin
dipyridamole (Persantine)
ticlopidine (Ticlid)—an investigational agent

Thrombolytic Enzymes

Anticoagulant drugs are not effective in dissolving clots that have already formed. Instead, thrombolytic enzymes are used to lyse the thrombi that obstruct coronary or pulmonary arteries. Thrombolytic enzymes act by converting plasminogen to plasmin. Plasmin (also known as fibrinolysin) is an enzyme which breaks apart (or lyses) fibrin and therefore is able to dissolve blood clots.

Thrombolytic enzyme drugs are always given intravenously and include:

alteplase (Activase)
anistreplase (APSAC, Eminase)
streptokinase (Kabikinase, Streptase)
urokinase (Abbokinase)

Note: The ending *-ase* is common to both the generic and trade names of thrombolytic enzymes; *-ase* is a suffix meaning *enzyme*.

Miscellaneous Drugs

cryoprecipitate   A plasma extract prepared by freezing and slow thawing of plasma, it contains concentrated amounts of clotting factor VIII, von Willebrand factor, and fibrinogen.

protamine sulfate. By binding with heparin to neutralize its anticoagulant effects, this drug's only therapeutic purpose is to treat heparin overdose or reverse the effects of heparin administered during open heart surgery with cardiopulmonary bypass.

vitamin K (AquaMEPHYTON, Mephyton, Synkayvite). A coagulant drug used to restore normal blood clotting time in patients who have had an overdose of anti-coagulants other than heparin. Also given prophylactically to newborns to prevent hemorrhage.

REVIEW QUESTIONS

1. Describe the difference between the therapeutic action of anticoagulants and that of thrombolytic enzymes.
2. What drug is used to reverse the effects of heparin?

18

Pulmonary Drugs

Respiratory diseases such as asthma, chronic obstructive pulmonary disease (COPD), and emphysema require medication to treat chronic and acute symptoms as well as prevent acute attacks. Aside from the antibiotics used to treat respiratory infections, there are two main classes of drugs prescribed to treat pulmonary diseases. These include bronchodilators and corticosteroids. The drugs used to treat tuberculosis will also be discussed.

Bronchodilators

Bronchodilators relax the smooth muscle that surrounds the bronchi, thereby increasing air flow. This dilatation of the bronchi is due either to stimulation of $beta_2$ receptors in the smooth muscle of the bronchi, the release of epinephrine which itself stimulates $beta_2$ receptors, or to inhibition of acetylcholine at cholinergic receptor sites in the smooth muscle. Some bronchodilators are given orally; some are given intravenously; some are prescribed as a solution in a dispenser (inhaler) with a special mouthpiece. The dispenser nebulizes the medicine and automatically injects a premeasured dose into the lungs as the patient inhales through the mouth. The prescribed dosage for these **metered-dose inhalers** is in numbers of puffs.

Bronchodilators administered through inhalers include:
> albuterol (Proventil, Ventolin)
> bitolterol (Tornalate)
> epinephrine (Bronkaid Mist, Primatene Mist)
> fenoterol HBr (Berotec)—an investigational drug
> ipratropium (Atrovent)
> isoetharine (Bronkometer, Bronkosol)
> isoproterenol (Isuprel, Medihaler-Iso)
> metaproterenol (Alupent, Metaprel)
> pirbuterol (Maxair)
> terbutaline (Brethaire)

Bronchodilators given orally include:
> albuterol (Proventil, Ventolin)
> aminophylline (Somophyllin)
> ephedrine

dyphylline (Lufyllin)
isoproterenol (Isuprel)
metaproterenol (Alupent, Metaprel)
oxtriphylline (Choledyl)
terbutaline (Brethine, Bricanyl)
theophylline (Bronkodyl, Constant-T, Duraphyl, Elixophyllin, Quibron,
     Respbid, Slo-bid Gyrocaps, Slo-Phyllin Gyrocaps,
     Somophyllin, Sustaire, Theo-24, Theobid, Theo-Dur
     Sprinkle, Theolair, Theophyl, Theovent)
Bronchodilators given I.V. include:
aminophylline
dyphylline (Lufyllin)
epinephrine (Adrenalin)
theophylline

DID YOU KNOW? Terbutaline under the trade name Bricanyl is also given
to stop premature labor contractions. It does this by stimulating beta$_2$ receptors in uterine smooth muscle, producing relaxation.

Combination Products

The following oral drugs combine two different bronchodilators and other
ingredients.

Bronkaid (theophylline and ephedrine and guaifenesin [an expectorant])
Marax (theophylline and ephedrine and hydroxyzine [Vistaril]–an anti-
     anxiety drug used to counteract the stimulant effects of ephedrine)
Primatene (theophylline and ephedrine)
Tedral (theophylline and ephedrine and phenobarbital [a sedative to counter-
     act the effects of ephedrine])

Corticosteroids

Corticosteroids reduce inflammation and tissue edema. They cannot provide
bronchodilation and so are always used in conjunction with the bronchodilators
described previously. Their use is prophylactic, and they are not effective during
acute attacks of bronchospasm. These drugs are given by inhaler, and the dosage
is prescribed as a number of puffs.

beclomethasone (Beclovent, Vanceril)
dexamethasone (Decadron Respihaler)
flunisolide (AeroBid)
triamcinolone (Azmacort)

Mast Cell Inhibitors

Mast cell inhibitors act to stabilize the membrane of mast cells and prevent the
release of histamine. This prevents the bronchospasm in patients with bronchial

asthma that is triggered by allergies. These drugs are not effective in treating acute attacks and are taken continuously for a prophylactic effect. Note: Cromolyn is given by nebulizer or by a special device called a **Spinhaler turbo-inhaler** which punctures the capsule and allows the powdered drug within to be inhaled. The other two drugs are investigational and can be given orally.

cromolyn (Intal)

ketotifen (Zaditen)—an investigational drug

nedocromil (Tilade)—an investigational drug

Antituberculosis Drugs

Tuberculosis is caused by *Mycobacterium tuberculosis,* a gram-positive rod which is resistant to antibiotics that are usually effective against gram-positive bacteria. Continuous therapy with some combination of the antituberculosis drugs listed below is usually necessary to complete treatment.

ethambutol (Myambutol)

isoniazid (INH, Nydrazid)

pyrazinamide

rifampin (Rifadin, Rimactane)

HISTORICAL NOTE: The microbiologist Selman Waksman (who discovered the antibiotic neomycin, the chemotherapy drug actinomycin D, and coined the term *antibiotic*) was a professor at Rutgers University where he studied soil bacteria. He was looking for a drug which was effective against tuberculosis, as the newly discovered wonder drug penicillin was not, unfortunately. He and his students examined 10,000 different soil samples looking for a substance that could kill tuberculosis. They examined a clump of dirt taken from the throat of a sick chicken. On it was growing the mold that would be found to destroy the tuberculosis bacteria. They called it *streptomycin.* Shortly before their discovery, however, a financial officer at Rutgers had suggested Waksman be fired to cut down on expenses, as his work was obscure and his research would never repay the money invested in it. After the discovery of streptomycin, he was offered ten million dollars which he turned over to Rutgers where, at his suggestion, they built a microbiology laboratory. Eventually, tuberculosis developed resistance to streptomycin, and it was replaced by the newer antitubercular drugs described above.

Antihistamines, antitussives, and expectorants are discussed in Chapter 19.

Miscellaneous Drugs

acetylcysteine (Mucomyst)   Used to treat very thick mucus secretions found in patients with cystic fibrosis and chronic pulmonary diseases such as emphysema, this drug dissolves the chemical bonds of mucoproteins and thins the mucus so that it can be expectorated.

DID YOU KNOW? Acetylcysteine (Mucomyst) is used as an antidote for acetaminophen (Tylenol) overdose. It acts to protect the liver, the main site of symptoms of toxicity from acetaminophen overdose.

---

bovine surfactant extract (Survanta)   This natural surfactant derived from ground up cows' lungs is used to supplement low levels of natural surfactant in the lungs of premature infants suffering from respiratory distress syndrome (RDS), also known as hyaline membrane disease. Surfactant maintains surface tension to prevent the lungs from collapsing with each breath. It is administered via an endotracheal tube.

colfosceril palmitate (Exosurf)   An investigational drug, this synthetic surfactant is used to supplement low levels of natural surfactant in the lungs of premature infants suffering from respiratory distress syndrome (RDS), also known as hyaline membrane disease. Surfactant maintains surface tension to prevent the lungs from collapsing with each breath. It is administered via an endotracheal tube.

diuretics   Used specifically to treat the pulmonary edema which results from left-sided congestive heart failure. See Chapter 12.

REVIEW QUESTIONS

1. Bronchodilators can be administered via what three routes?
2. Terbutaline is a bronchodilator and also has been used to stop premature labor contractions. True or False?
3. Corticosteroids can be inhaled to provide relief from an acute asthma attack. True or False?
4. Mucomyst is used to treat patients with cystic fibrosis and acetaminophen overdose. True or False?

SPELLING TIPS

- Azmacort, used to treat asthma (Note how differently this sound-alike drug is spelled from the disease.)
- Bronkaid, Bronkometer, Bronkosol (Spelled with a *k*, not *ch*.)
- Slo-Phyllin (difficult to spell because it is alternately pronounced as either "sa-law'fa-lin" or "slow-fillin").
- AeroBid (Unusual due to internal capitalization.)

19

Ear, Nose, and Throat (ENT) Drugs

ENT drugs are prescribed for various conditions of the ears, nose, and throat ranging from swimmer's ear to nasal polyps to coughs and colds to seasonal or allergic rhinitis. ENT drugs comprise several distinct classes of drugs, including decongestants, antihistamines, antitussives, expectorants, corticosteroids, and antibiotics, all of which are discussed below.

> DID YOU KNOW? Most people contract one to two colds per year. There are over 120 different viruses that cause colds, not to mention bacterial sources. The common cold is considered the single most expensive illness in the United States in terms of time lost from work and school. No medication is currently available to cure the common cold or shorten its duration; available drugs merely provide temporary relief of various symptoms until the cold has run its course.

Decongestants

Decongestants act as vasoconstrictors which reduce blood flow to edematous tissues in the nose, sinuses, and pharynx; they achieve this vasoconstriction by stimulating alpha receptors in these tissues. Decongestants decrease the swelling of mucous membranes, alleviate nasal stuffiness, allow secretions to drain, and help to unclog the eustachian tubes. Decongestants are commonly prescribed for colds and allergies. They can be administered topically as nose drops or nasal sprays, or can be taken orally. Decongestants are often combined with antihistamines in cold remedies.

Decongestant drugs include:

ephedrine
oxymetazoline (Afrin, Duration)
phenylephrine (Neo-Synephrine)
phenylpropanolamine
pseudoephedrine (Afrinol, Sudafed)
xylometazoline (Otrivin)

Antihistamines

Antihistamines exert their therapeutic effect by blocking **histamine (H_1) receptors** in the nose, throat, and eyes. Histamine is released by the antibody-antigen complex that occurs during allergic reactions. Histamine causes vasodilation which allows blood vessels and tissues to become engorged, swollen, and red. Histamine also irritates these tissues directly, causing pain and itching. Antihistamines block the action of histamine at the H_1 receptors. This helps to dry up secretions, shrink edematous mucous membranes, and decrease itching and redness. A significant side effect of early antihistamines was drowsiness; however, newer antihistamines such as terfenadine (Seldane) and astemizole (Hismanal) have a different chemical structure that does not cross the blood-brain barrier to produce drowsiness.

Antihistamine drugs include:

    astemizole (Hismanal)
    brompheniramine (Dimetane)
    chlorpheniramine (Chlor-Trimeton)
    clemastine (Tavist)
    diphenhydramine (Benadryl)
    loratadine (Claritin)—an investigational drug
    terfenadine (Seldane)

Antihistamines are effective only in treating allergic reactions which release histamine. They are not effective in treating the common cold. Although symptoms of allergies and colds are similar, there is no release of histamine with the common cold. Nevertheless, pharmaceutical manufacturers continue to combine antihistamines with decongestants in cold remedies.

Antitussive Drugs

Antitussives act to decrease coughing by suppressing the cough center in the brain. Their main purpose is to stop nonproductive dry coughs. They are not prescribed for productive coughs which are generating sputum. Some antitussives are narcotics, such as codeine and hydrocodone; these are prescription schedule drugs. Over-the-counter antitussives contain the non-narcotic dextromethorphan. Antitussives are incorporated into many cold remedies.

    codeine
    dextromethorphan (Sucrets, Pertussin)
    hydrocodone (Hycodan)

Many over-the-counter products with varying ingredients signify the presence of dextromethorphan by including *DM* in the trade name (example: Robitussin-DM).

Expectorants

Expectorants act to reduce the viscosity or thickness of sputum so that patients can more easily cough it up. Expectorants are prescribed only for productive coughs.

    guaifenesin (Robitussin)
    terpin hydrate

Combination Drugs

The following trade name drugs contain various combinations of decongestants, antihistamines, antitussives, and expectorants as well as the pain relievers, acetaminophen and ibuprofen.

Decongestant/antihistamine combination

Actifed	Naldecon
Allerest	Novahistine
Benylin	Ornade
Contac	Rondec
Deconamine	Triaminic
Dimetapp	Trinalin Repetabs
Drixoral	

Decongestant/pain reliever combination
CoAdvil
Dristan
Sine-Aid

Antihistamine/pain reliever combination
Percogesic

Miscellaneous combinations
Comtrex—decongestant, antihistamine, non-narcotic antitussive, and pain reliever
Entex LA—decongestant and expectorant
Formula 44—antihistamine and non-narcotic antitussive
Hycomine—decongestant, antihistamine, narcotic antitussive, and pain reliever
NyQuil—decongestant, antitussive, and pain reliever
Pertussin—decongestant and non-narcotic antitussive
Phenergan with Codeine—antihistamine and narcotic antitussive
Tussi-Organidin—expectorant and narcotic antitussive

Corticosteroids

Corticosteroids act by inhibiting many aspects of the body's inflammatory response, including decreasing capillary dilatation, decreasing numbers of local white blood cells, and decreasing edema. Corticosteroids have no antihistamine effect and are not prescribed for mild allergies. Allergic reactions producing a body rash and itching may be treated with oral corticosteroids. Corticosteroids have no effect on the common cold. They are, however, effective when administered intranasally to topically treat nasal polyps and nonallergic (vasomotor) rhinitis. Intranasal corticosteroids include:

beclomethasone (Beconase, Vancenase)
dexamethasone (Decadron Turbinaire)
flunisolide (Nasalide)

Triamcinolone is a corticosteroid paste which is applied topically to the mouth to treat ulcers and inflammation.

triamcinolone (Kenalog in Orabase)

Antibiotics

Antibiotics are not effective in treating the common cold when it is caused by a virus; however, they are prescribed for colds caused by bacterial infections, particularly streptococci. They may also be prescribed prophylactically for patients with viral colds to prevent superimposed bacterial infections. See Chapter 27 for a complete discussion of oral antibiotics.

Antibiotic solutions may be prescribed for topical application in the ears to treat external otitis media and other infections.

    chloramphenicol (Chloromycetin Otic)

Corticosteroid and antibiotic drugs are often combined in a single solution for topical application in the ear. They include:

    Coly-Mycin S Otic (colistin, hydrocortisone, neomycin)

    Cortisporin Otic (hydrocortisone, neomycin, polymyxin B)

    Otobiotic Otic (hydrocortisone, polymyxin B)

Antifungal Agents

Yeasts, which are closely related to fungi, grow easily in the warm, dark environment of the mouth, particularly in immunocompromised patients. Topical drugs used to treat oral yeast infections caused by *Candida albicans* include:

    clotrimazole (Mycelex)

    ketoconazole (Nizoral)

    nystatin (Mycostatin, Nilstat)

Candida albicans infections are alternatively known as oral candidiasis, monilia, or thrush. The above drugs are applied topically as a solution (for **"swish and swallow"**) or supplied as a **troche** (a lozenge). Nizoral is also available as an oral tablet which acts systemically.

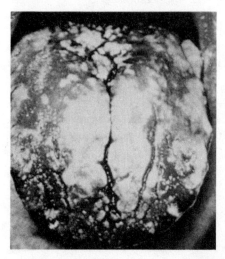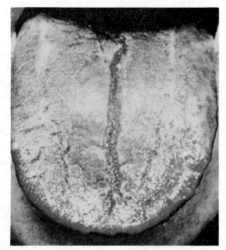

FIGURE 19-1

Severe oral thrush before and after treatment with Nizoral. Photo courtesy of Kallir, Phillips, Ross, Inc., New York.

Motion Sickness Drugs

For drugs that control dizziness associated with overstimulation of the inner ear, see Antiemetics, Chapter 13, page 66.

Miscellaneous Drugs

Anbesol   Topical over-the-counter anesthetic solution for the mouth and throat.

benzocaine (Auralgan Otic)   Topical anesthetic solution for the ear.

Cepacol   Over-the-counter throat lozenge containing a topical anesthetic.

Cerumenex   Topical agent which softens hardened ear wax (cerumen) and allows it to be flushed from the ear.

Chloraseptic   Over-the-counter throat spray containing a topical anesthetic.

cocaine   Topical anesthetic and vasoconstrictor used during examinations and operations on the nose.

DID YOU KNOW? Cocaine addicts who sniff the powder often have intranasal ulcers and can even develop a perforated nasal septum. This is due to the powerful topical vasoconstrictor action of cocaine which, when applied frequently, actually causes sloughing of the mucous membranes.

---

cromolyn (Nasalcrom)   A mast cell inhibitor which prevents the release of histamine from mast cells, this drug comes as a nasal spray and is used prophylactically to prevent allergy symptoms.

lidocaine (Xylocaine)   Prescription topical anesthetic for mouth ulcers and denture pain.

Ocean Mist   A nasal moistener for dried mucous membranes.

silver nitrate   A cauterizing agent on an applicator stick used to cauterize superficial blood vessels causing repeated nosebleeds.

Tessalon Perles   A prescription anesthetic, taken orally, which acts only on the respiratory tract to relieve intractable, nonproductive coughing. A non-narcotic antitussive.

DID YOU KNOW? Vicks VapoRub, a topical ointment sometimes applied to the chest of persons with colds, contains eucalyptus oil and spirits of turpentine.

REVIEW QUESTIONS

1. State your position as a consumer advocate on the cost-effectiveness of including an antihistamine ingredient in an over-the-counter cold remedy.
2. What is the difference between the therapeutic action of antitussive drugs and expectorants?

20

Ophthalmic Drugs

Ophthalmic drugs may be applied topically to treat superficial infection or inflammation of the cornea and surrounding tissues, and to treat glaucoma; other ophthalmic drugs are taken systemically for severe infection or inflammation in the interior of the eye. All drugs intended for topical application in the eye are specially formulated in a base solution that is physiologically similar to fluids in the eye so as not to damage delicate eye tissues.

Antibiotics

Used to treat superficial infections of the cornea, conjunctivae, eyelids, and tear ducts, topical antibiotics prevent bacteria from maintaining their cell wall. Antibiotics are not effective against viral infections. Ophthalmic antibiotics are dispensed as ointments or solutions. Topical antibiotics for the eye include:

bacitracin
chloramphenicol (Chloromycetin, Chloroptic, Ophthochlor)
chlortetracycline (Aureomycin)
erythromycin (Ilotycin)
gentamicin (Garamycin, Genoptic)
tetracycline (Achromycin)
tobramycin (Tobrex)

Ophthalmic products containing several topical antibiotics together include:

Mycitracin Ophthalmic (bacitracin, neomycin, polymyxin B)
Neosporin Ophthalmic (neomycin, polymyxin B)
Polysporin (bacitracin, polymyxin B)

Oral antibiotics given systemically for severe eye infections are discussed in Chapter 27, pages 141-145.

Most states either recommend or require the use of a topical anti-infective agent to be applied to the eyes of newborn infants to prevent infection and possible blindness from gonorrhea (contacted as the baby's head moves through the infected birth canal). Anti-infectives used for this purpose include:

silver nitrate
erythromycin (Ilotycin)
tetracycline (Achromycin)

Although silver nitrate has been commonly used for years and is the least expensive, it has several drawbacks: conjunctival irritation/swelling which may interfere with mother-child bonding, and ineffectiveness in preventing eye infections from *Chlamydia* (another sexually transmitted disease). Neither erythromycin nor tetracycline has these limitations.

Antiviral Drugs

Antiviral drugs act by inhibiting viral DNA reproduction. The herpes simplex virus, types 1 and 2, causes conjunctivitis and corneal ulcers. Topical antiviral drugs for the eye include:

idoxuridine (Herplex)
trifluridine (Viroptic)
vidarabine (Vira-A)

Corticosteroids

Corticosteroid drugs are used topically in the eye to treat the inflammation that results from trauma or contact with chemicals. These drugs include:

dexamethasone (Decadron, Maxidex)
prednisolone (Inflamase, Pred Forte)

Combination corticosteroids and antibiotic drugs include:

Maxitrol (dexamethasone, neomycin, polymyxin B)
NeoDecadron (dexamethasone, neomycin)
Ophthocort (hydrocortisone, chloramphenicol, polymyxin B)

Topical Anesthetics

Topical anesthetic drugs are used in the eye to facilitate examination and for short procedures such as foreign body or suture removal. These drugs include:

proparacaine (Ophthaine, Ophthetic)
tetracaine (Pontocaine)

Drugs for Glaucoma

Glaucoma is a disease whose presenting symptom is increased intraocular pressure. If untreated, it can lead to blindness. Drugs for glaucoma act either by decreasing the amount of aqueous humor circulating in the anterior and posterior chambers, or by constricting the pupil (miotic action) so as to open the angle of contact between the iris and the trabecular meshwork, allowing the aqueous humor to flow freely.

Direct-acting miotics cause pupillary constriction by stimulating the iris muscle around the pupil to contract. Miotic drugs used to treat glaucoma include:

acetylcholine (Miochol)
carbachol (Miostat)
pilocarpine (Ocusert Pilo, Pilagan, Pilocar)

Other miotic drugs act by inhibiting cholinesterase, an enzyme which normally destroys acetylcholine. The increased levels of acetylcholine then result in miosis.

Miotic drugs which act in this way include:
>   demecarium (Humorsol)
>   echothiophate iodide
>   isofluorophate (Floropryl)
>   physostigmine

Other topical drugs which do not constrict the pupil but increase the outflow of aqueous humor include:
>   apraclonidine (Iopidine)
>   epinephrine (Epifrin, Epitrate, Eppy/N)
>   dipivefrin (Propine)

Another group of drugs used to treat glaucoma includes topical beta blockers. They act by blocking the production of aqueous humor to decrease intraocular pressure. They have no effect on pupil size and therefore do not cause the blurred vision or night blindness associated with other miotics which constrict and fix the pupil. Topical beta blocker drugs given for glaucoma include:
>   betaxolol (Betoptic)
>   levobunolol (Betagan)
>   timolol (Timoptic)

Mydriatics

This group of topical drugs is used to dilate the pupil (mydriasis) and paralyze the muscles of accommodation (cycloplegia) of the iris. They do this by blocking the action of acetylcholine which normally tends to constrict the pupil. Mydriatic drugs are used to prepare the eye for internal examination and also to treat inflammatory conditions of the iris and uveal tract. Topical mydriatic drugs include:
>   atropine
>   cyclopentolate (Cyclogyl)
>   homatropine
>   scopolamine
>   tropicamide (Mydriacyl)

DID YOU KNOW? The belladonna plant was the original source of atropine and scopolamine. Belladonna means *beautiful lady* in Italian. "Sixteenth century Italian women . . . squeezed the berries of these plants into their eyes to widen and brighten them."

>   Michael C. Gerald, *Pharmacology: An Introduction to Drugs,* 2d ed.
>   (Englewood Cliffs, N.J.: Prentice-Hall, 1981), p. 149

Scopolamine is also used for motion sickness, but has a side effect of blurred vision from paralysis of the muscles of accommodation around the pupil.

Miscellaneous Drugs

Adsorbonac A hypertonic sodium chloride solution applied topically to help reduce corneal edema following cataract surgery and other procedures.

alpha-chymotrypsin See *chymotrypsin*.

balanced salt solution See *BSS*.

botulinum toxin type A (Oculinum) Derived from a culture of the same bacteria which cause botulism (food poisoning), this drug is injected into eye muscles where it paralyzes the muscle fibers and allows them to lengthen. It is used to treat blepharospasm and may, in the future, replace surgical correction of strabismus.

BSS An abbreviation for balanced salt solution, an intraocular irrigant of physiologic saline solution used during eye surgery to irrigate and protect the eye.

bupivacaine (Marcaine) A local anesthetic given by retrobulbar injection to produce anesthesia and akinesia (temporary paralysis) of the eye muscles before surgery.

chymotrypsin (Catarase, Zolyse) An enzyme used to lyse fibers which hold the lens in place prior to removing the lens during intraocular surgery.

cromolyn (Opticrom) A mast cell inhibitor which prevents the release of histamine from mast cells. This topical drug specifically prevents allergic symptoms in the eye.

fluorescein A yellow water-based dye which shows green under fluorescent light, this drug is used to point out corneal abrasions and ulcers caused by foreign bodies or ill-fitting contact lenses.

flurbiprofen (Ocufen) An anti-inflammatory agent used to prevent contraction of the pupil during surgery and prevent postoperative edema.

Lacrisert A pellet inserted into the conjunctival sac which continuously releases artificial tears to lubricate the eye.

Liquifilm Topical artificial tears solution for dry, irritated eyes.

sodium hyaluronate (Amvisc, Healon, Viscoat) Injected into the anterior chamber of the eye during intraocular surgery, this drug protects the eye, keeps the anterior chamber expanded, and replaces lost aqueous humor.

tolrestat (Alredase) Used to treat diabetic retinopathy, this investigational drug acts to inhibit the accumulation of sorbitol in eye tissues, a substance which causes cellular damage. Sorbitol is produced from glucose; excess quantities from the hyperglycemia of diabetes can damage the eye.

REVIEW QUESTIONS

1. Discuss the use of silver nitrate versus erythromycin to prevent newborns from having eye infections from gonorrhea.
2. What advantage do beta blockers have over other miotic drugs used to treat glaucoma?
3. What class of drugs is used to prepare the eye for examination?

21

Endocrine Drugs

The endocrine system consists of many glands which secrete hormones into the bloodstream. Those of major importance in drug therapy include the thyroid gland which secretes thyroxine (T_4) and triiodothyronine (T_3); the pituitary gland which secretes growth hormone and vasopressin; and the adrenal gland whose cortex secretes aldosterone and corticosteroids. When these glands malfunction due to disease processes, they may release either a decreased or increased level of hormone. Drugs may then be given either as supplements to normalize hormone levels or to counteract increased hormone levels.

Thyroid Gland Drugs

Thyroid supplements are used to treat hypothyroidism. These drugs are obtained either from natural sources such as desiccated (dried) ground animal thyroid glands or may be synthetically manufactured.

These thyroid supplements contain both T_3 and T_4:
> desiccated thyroid
> liotrix (Euthroid, Thyrolar)
> thyroglobulin (Proloid)

This supplement contains only T_3:
> liothyronine (Cytomel)

This supplement contains only T_4:
> levothyroxine (Synthroid)

Drugs used to treat hyperthyroidism act by inhibiting the production of T_3 and T_4 in the thyroid gland. These drugs include:
> propylthiouracil
> methimazole (Tapazole)
> radioactive sodium iodide 131

Pituitary Gland Drugs

The pituitary gland secretes growth hormone. Decreased levels of this hormone inhibit skeletal growth in children. Drugs used as replacement therapy include:
> somatrem (Protropin)
> somatropin (Humatrope)

The pituitary gland also secretes vasopressin which inhibits the excretion of water by the kidneys. Vasopressin is also known as ADH or antidiuretic hormone because of its action as described. A lack of ADH results in diabetes insipidus. Drugs used as replacement therapy include:

> desmopressin (DDAVP)
> lypressin (Diapid)
> vasopressin (Pitressin)

DID YOU KNOW? Desmopressin has also been used to treat bed-wetting. Studies have shown that many patients who habitually bed wet have low levels of ADH. Therefore desmopressin (DDAVP) is given in a nasal spray as replacement therapy.

Adrenal Gland Drugs

The adrenal gland secretes many hormones, but one of particular interest which exhibits low levels due to the disease process of Addison disease is that of aldosterone. Drugs used as replacement therapy include:

> desoxycorticosterone (Percorten)
> fludrocortisone (Florinef)

The adrenal cortex also secretes hydrocortisone and cortisone, powerful anti-inflammatory hormones. These and other synthetic anti-inflammatory agents are known as corticosteroids. They are commonly prescribed to systemically inhibit inflammatory reactions throughout the body. These oral corticosteroid drugs include:

> betamethasone (Celestone)
> cortisone
> dexamethasone (Decadron)
> hydrocortisone (Cortef, Hydrocortone, Solu-Cortef)
> methylprednisolone (Depo-Medrol, Medrol, Solu-Medrol)
> paramethasone (Haldrone)
> prednisolone (Delta-Cortef)
> prednisone (Deltasone)
> triamcinolone (Aristocort, Kenacort, Kenalog)

For the use of topical steroid drugs, see Chapter 11; steroids for the GI tract, Chapter 13; steroids in orthopedics, Chapter 14; steroids for the respiratory tract, Chapter 18; steroids for the ENT system, Chapter 19.

HISTORICAL NOTE: A researcher at the Mayo Clinic was attempting to identify hormones in the adrenal gland. He located five substances which he called Substances A, B, C, D, and E. To obtain only two ounces of Substance E, he had to grind 300,000 pounds of cattle adrenal glands. In 1941 the United States received an intelligence report that Germany was giving adrenal gland extracts to its pilots to enable them to fly at high altitudes. Although this report was false, it provided financial backing for adrenal gland research. Substance E later became known as *cortisone*.

22

Antidiabetic Drugs

Diabetes mellitus results when the pancreas fails to produce any insulin (type I diabetes mellitus) or produces too little (type II diabetes mellitus). Type I diabetes mellitus is also known as insulin-dependent diabetes mellitus or juvenile-onset diabetes mellitus. Type II diabetes mellitus is also known as non-insulin-dependent diabetes mellitus or adult-onset diabetes mellitus. Type I must always be treated with subcutaneously injected insulin; type II may be treated with insulin or, more commonly, with diet and/or oral antidiabetic drugs.

Insulin is secreted by beta cells in the islets of Langerhans in the pancreas. This hormone plays an essential role in sugar metabolism.

HISTORICAL NOTE: Insulin was first isolated in the 1920s. Until that time, diabetic patients were kept on an extremely low calorie diet (often to the point of starvation)—the only treatment known. The term *insulin* was taken from the Latin word *insula* meaning *island,* a reference to the islets of Langerhans. The first insulin injections were thick and muddy brown in color due to impurities from their source: ground up beef and pork pancreas.

Insulin is derived from beef or pork pancreas or from human insulin (which overcomes the potential for allergic reactions). Human insulin is genetically produced using recombinant DNA techniques. Regardless of the original source, all insulins are classified according to how quickly they act (which depends on the size of the insulin crystal) and how many hours their therapeutic action continues (which is lengthened by the addition of protamine).

Rapid-acting insulins include:
  regular (Regular Iletin, Humulin BR, Humulin R, Novolin R, Velosulin)
  semilente (Semilente Iletin)
Intermediate-acting insulins include:
  NPH (NPH Iletin, Humulin N, Insulatard NPH, Novolin N)
  lente (Lente Iletin, Humulin L, Novolin L)
Long-acting insulins include:
  protamine zinc (PZI)
  ultralente (Ultralente Iletin, Humulin U)

Mixtures of 70% NPH and 30% regular insulin are also available as:
Humulin 70/30
Mixtard 70/30
Novolin 70/30
Note: The trade name for all human genetically produced insulins is Humulin.

Insulin is given subcutaneously once or twice a day at various sites on the arms, thighs, or abdomen. It can also be administered directly into the bloodstream by an implantable computerized insulin pump. Insulin dosages are always measured in units.

Oral Antidiabetic Agents

A patient with type II diabetes mellitus has a pancreas which is still producing limited amounts of insulin. With diet control and weight loss, this amount of insulin may be sufficient. If not, an oral antidiabetic agent may be ordered. Contrary to popular opinion, these drugs are not insulin but act to stimulate the pancreas to produce more insulin. Oral antidiabetic agents are not effective for a patient with type I diabetes mellitus whose pancreas no longer produces any insulin. Oral antidiabetic agents include:

acetohexamide (Dymelor)
chlorpropamide (Diabinese)
glipizide (Glucotrol)
glyburide (Diaßeta, Micronase)
tolazamide (Tolinase)
tolbutamide (Orinase)

REVIEW QUESTIONS

1. Oral antidiabetic agents contain a special kind of insulin which can be taken by mouth. True or False?
2. The trade name for genetically produced insulin is Humulin. True or False?

SPELLING TIPS

- Diaßeta (The symbol ß is the Greek letter beta, a reference to the beta cells of the pancreas which produce insulin.)

23

Obstetric and Gynecologic Drugs

Drugs used to treat women with obstetric and gynecologic problems include drugs for infertility and vaginal infections, drugs which stimulate or suppress labor contractions, drugs which correct menstrual disorders and endometriosis, estrogen replacement therapy, and prophylactically prescribed birth control agents.

Drugs for Infertility

Although surgical intervention plays an important part in reversing some types of female infertility, drug therapy for infertility is also important and includes ovulation stimulating agents. These drugs are not appropriate for patients with blocked fallopian tubes or other mechanical problems requiring surgical intervention. Ovulation stimulating agents act by stimulating the pituitary gland to release luteinizing hormone (LH) and follicle stimulating hormone (FSH) which help the ovary prepare and release mature eggs. These drugs also aid in the formation of the corpus luteum which secretes progesterone to maintain the pregnancy if the ovum is fertilized. Ovulation stimulating drugs may cause several mature eggs to be released, resulting in multiple births. These drugs include:

clomiphene (Clomid)
human chorionic gonadotropin (HCG or hCG, Follutein, Pregnyl, A.P.L.)
menotropins (Pergonal)
urofollitropin (Metrodin)

Note: Clomid can be used alone, but menotropins and urofollitropin must be given concurrently with HCG to achieve a complete therapeutic effect.

DID YOU KNOW? The drugs menotropins and urofollitropin are manufactured from the urine of postmenopausal women.

Drugs Used During Pregnancy

Few drugs are prescribed during pregnancy, particularly in the first trimester, due to the increased risk of birth defects (see references to thalidomide, page 9). However, antibiotics for infections and drugs to maintain good health (such as insulin or heart medications) as well as prenatal vitamins and iron may be given.

Uterine Relaxants

Premature delivery greatly increases morbidity and mortality in infants. Premature labor contractions may be inhibited by using uterine relaxing drugs which act on beta$_2$ receptors in the smooth muscle of the uterus to effect relaxation. These drugs decrease both the frequency and strength of contractions.

      ritodrine (Yutopar)

      terbutaline (Bricanyl)

DID YOU KNOW? Terbutaline also acts on beta$_2$ receptors in the smooth muscle around the bronchi to produce bronchodilation. It is used to treat bronchial asthma and is marketed under the trade names Brethaire and Brethine.

Uterine Stimulants

Women who are in labor and whose membranes have ruptured may be given the uterine stimulant oxytocin if their uterine contractions are too weak to effect delivery. Oxytocin is normally produced by the pituitary gland and directly stimulates the uterus by binding to special oxytocin receptors in the uterine muscle. Oxytocin increases both the frequency and strength of uterine contractions. Oxytocin is not indicated when prolonged labor is due to cephalopelvic disproportion.

      oxytocin (Pitocin)

Postpartum bleeding is due to too great a degree of uterine relaxation which results in increased bleeding at the site of placental separation. Uterine stimulating drugs are also used to treat this condition. These drugs include:

      oxytocin (Pitocin)

      ergonovine (Ergotrate)

      methylergonovine (Methergine)

Drugs Used to Treat Endometriosis

Endometriosis is caused by uterine tissue which implants within the pelvic cavity and on the ovaries and other organs. It continues to remain sensitive to hormonal influence, secreting blood when the uterus begins menstruation. Endometriosis causes pelvic pain, inflammation, and cyst formation. After using drugs to suppress the menstrual cycle for several months, endometrial implants may atrophy. Drugs used to treat endometriosis include:

      danazol (Danocrine)—oral administration

      nafarelin (Synarel)—administration by nasal spray

Oral Contraceptives

Birth control pills exert a hormonal influence to prevent pregnancy and are 95% effective if taken as directed. Most oral contraceptives contain a combination of estrogen and progesterone (or progestin) which is taken for 21 days. During the final seven days of the 28-day menstrual cycle, the patient may take no tablets, or seven sugar-filled tablets or sugar tablets with iron may be included in the pill case. Other oral contraceptives contain only progesterone.

IN DEPTH: Estrogen normally is secreted by the ovaries and causes the endometrium to proliferate. It also causes follicles to grow on the ovary and release mature ova during ovulation. Progesterone is first secreted by the corpus luteum in the middle of the menstrual cycle. If an ovum is fertilized, the corpus luteum continues to secrete progesterone to prepare the endometrium to accept the fertilized egg. If the ovum is not fertilized, the corpus luteum disintegrates, thus stopping progesterone production. When this happens, the uterine lining sloughs off in the process of menstruation.

Combination oral contraceptives. Combination oral contraceptives containing both estrogen and progesterone are divided into three basic groups according to the relative amounts of progesterone and estrogen provided during each day of the menstrual cycle. These three basic groups of combination oral contraceptives include monophasics, biphasics, and triphasics.

The **monophasic** group of oral combination contraceptives provides the same fixed amounts of progesterone and estrogen in every tablet for each day of the 21-day segment. The amounts of progesterone and estrogen are designated by two numbers following the trade name drugs. Example: Norinyl 1+50 contains 1 mg of progesterone and 50 mcg of estrogen in every daily tablet. Because there have been increased side effects (particularly thrombophlebitis) associated with higher estrogen dosages, a physician may elect to prescribe Norinyl 1+35 which contains 1 mg of progesterone and 35 mcg of estrogen in every daily tablet.

Demulen 1/50	Demulen 1/35
Loestrin 1.5/30	Loestrin 1/20
Norinyl 1+50	Norinyl 1+35
Norlestrin 1/50	Norlestrin 2.5/50
Ortho-Novum 1/50	Ortho-Novum 1/35
Ovcon-50	Ovcon-35
Ovral	Lo/Ovral

The **biphasic** group of oral combination contraceptives provides a fixed amount of estrogen in every tablet for each day of the 21-day segment; the amount of progesterone is fixed in the first half of the cycle but then increases in the second half of the cycle. The change is designated by two numbers following the trade name drugs. Example: Ortho-Novum 10/11 provides 0.5 mg of progesterone and 35 mcg of estrogen in every tablet for the first 10 days segment; for the final 11 days, each tablet contains 1 mg of progesterone and 35 mcg of estrogen.

Nelova 10/11
Ortho-Novum 10/11

The **triphasic** group of oral combination contraceptives provides a fixed amount of estrogen on each day of the 21 days; the amount of progesterone increases or varies through the cycle. This is designated, at least in the case of Ortho-Novum, by the numbers 7/7/7 which show that the first seven tablets contain 0.5 mg of progesterone and 35 mcg of estrogen, the second seven tablets contain 1 mg of progesterone and 35 mcg of estrogen, and the last seven tablets of the 21-day segment contain 0.5 mg of progesterone and 35 mcg of estrogen.

> Ortho-Novum 7/7/7
> Tri-Levlen
> Tri-Norinyl
> Triphasil

Progesterone-only contraceptives. Contraceptives which contain only progesterone are slightly less effective in preventing pregnancy than combination contraceptives, particularly if the patient forgets to take even one daily tablet. However, the risks (particularly thrombophlebitis) and the side effects of estrogen therapy are avoided. Progesterone-only oral contraceptives include:

> Micronor
> Ovrette

Other progesterone-only contraceptives include Progestasert, which is inserted into the uterine cavity and is effective for one year, and Norplant, which is manufactured in six small silicone capsules that are implanted under the skin of the upper arm. Norplant is an effective contraceptive for five years.

Estrogen Replacement Therapy

As women enter menopause, the ovaries secrete decreasing amounts of estrogen. This can produce symptoms of vaginal dryness, hot flashes (due to vasodilation), and fatigue. Estrogen replacement therapy corrects the deficiency of this hormone. Estrogen may be given orally, by injection, or applied as a transdermal patch. A topical cream may be used to treat vaginal symptoms only.

> chlorotrianisene (Tace)
> conjugated estrogens (Premarin)
> esterified estrogens (Estratab, Menest)
> estradiol (Estrace, Estraderm)
> estradiol cypionate (Depo-Estradiol, Depogen)
> estropipate (Ogen)
> ethinyl estradiol (Estinyl)
> quinestrol (Estrovis)

Estrogen may also be combined with the antianxiety agent meprobamate to treat postmenopausal nervousness and depression in the trade name drugs **PMB** and **Menrium**.

Drugs to Treat Amenorrhea

Amenorrhea, the absence of menstruation, may be treated with drugs that stimulate the release of luteinizing hormone (LH) and follicle stimulating hormone (FSH) from the pituitary gland.

> gonadorelin (Lutrepulse)

Amenorrhea may also be treated with progesterone-like drugs which act directly on the tissues of the endometrium to produce menstruation. These drugs include:

> hydroxyprogesterone (Hylutin)

medroxyprogesterone (Provera)
norethindrone (Aygestin, Norlutate, Norlutin)

Drugs Used to Treat Dysmenorrhea

Painful menstrual cramps are caused by an increase in prostaglandins that cause the uterus to contract painfully. Prescription drugs which inhibit the action of prostaglandins have been specifically approved for the treatment of dysmenorrhea. These drugs include:

ibuprofen (Motrin)
ketoprofen (Orudis)
mefenamic acid (Ponstel)
naproxen (Naprosyn)

Note: Ibuprofen is the active ingredient in these over-the-counter drugs for menstrual cramps: Haltran, Midol, and Pamprin.

Drugs to Produce Abortion

When injected or given by suppository, large doses of certain prostaglandins can cause the uterus to contract strongly enough to spontaneously abort a fetus. These drugs are used to terminate a pregnancy.

carboprost (Hemabate)
dinoprost (Prostin F2 Alpha)
dinoprostone (Prostin E2)

DID YOU KNOW? While prostaglandin E2 (Prostin E2) is used to abort a fetus, prostaglandin E1 (alprostadil, Prostin VR) is used to save the lives of infants born with congenital heart defects. Prostin VR keeps open the ductus arteriosus which normally closes at birth so that these infants can maintain adequate oxygenation in spite of circulatory anomalies until surgical correction can be obtained.

Drugs to Treat Vaginal Infections

Vaginal infections and vaginitis are commonly caused by *Candida albicans* (a yeast), *Trichomonas vaginalis* (a flagellated parasite), and *Haemophilus vaginalis*, also known as *Gardnerella vaginalis* (a gram-negative rod).

Most drugs used to treat vaginal infections are applied topically and are manufactured in the form of creams/ointments, suppositories, or vaginal tablets. Drugs given orally are noted below.

Drugs used to treat candidal infections include:

butoconazole (Femstat)
clotrimazole (Gyne-Lotrimin, Mycelex-G)
miconazole (Monistat)
nystatin (Mycostatin, Nilstat)—also given orally
sulfanilamide (AVC)

terconazole (Terazol)
tioconazole (Vagistat)

Note: Many drugs used to treat candidal infections end in -*azole*. This ending signifies an antifungal drug. *Candida albicans* is a yeast, closely related to fungi and susceptible to many of the same drugs.

DID YOU KNOW? Nystatin was discovered in 1950 by two physicians who named the drug for their employer—the New York State Department of Health.

Drugs used to treat *Trichomonas vaginalis* infections include:
metronidazole (Flagyl) (given orally)
Drugs used to treat *Haemophilus* or *Gardnerella vaginalis* include:
ampicillin (Amcill, Omnipen, Polycillin)—given orally
metronidazole (Flagyl)—given orally
triple sulfa (Sultrin)—a sulfa anti-infective agent

Drugs for Pelvic Inflammatory Disease

Pelvic inflammatory disease involves widespread inflammation, scarring, and pain in the pelvic cavity. It is caused by sexually transmitted diseases as well as several other bacterial agents and is treated with systemic antibiotics, particularly doxycycline (Vibramycin). See the discussion of sexually transmitted diseases below and also antibiotics, Chapter 27.

Drugs for Sexually Transmitted Diseases (STDs)

Common sexually transmitted diseases (STDs) include gonorrhea, syphilis, chlamydia, and herpes.

Gonorrhea is caused by the gram-negative coccus *Neisseria gonorrhoeae*. Drugs used to treat gonorrhea include:
amoxicillin (Amoxil, Larotid)
ampicillin (Amcill, Omnipen, Polycillin, Principen, Totacillin)
bacampicillin (Spectrobid)
carbenicillin (Geopen, Pyopen)
cefoperazone (Cefobid)
ceforanide (Precef)
cefotaxime (Claforan)
cefotetan (Cefotan)
cefoxitin (Mefoxin)
cefuroxime (Zinacef)
ceftriaxone (Rocephin)
ciprofloxacin (Cipro)
demeclocycline (Declomycin)
doxycycline (Vibramycin)
erythromycin (E.E.S., E-Mycin, ERYC, Ilotycin)

      methacycline (Rondomycin)
      mezlocillin (Mezlin)
      minocycline (Minocin)
      penicillin G (Pentids, Wycillin)
      penicillin V (Pen-Vee K, V-Cillin K)
      piperacillin (Pipracil)
      tetracycline (Achromycin V, Sumycin)
      spectinomycin (Trobicin)

    Syphilis is caused by the gram-negative spirochete *Treponema pallidum.* Drugs used to treat syphilis include:

      penicillin G (Pentids, Wycillin)
      penicillin V (Pen-Vee K, V-Cillin K)

Penicillin is the drug of choice for treating syphilis, but for patients allergic to penicillin, these drugs may be used.

      demeclocycline (Declomycin)
      doxycycline (Vibramycin)
      erythromycin (E.E.S., E-Mycin, Eryc, Ilotycin)
      methacycline (Rondomycin)
      minocycline (Minocin)
      tetracycline (Achromycin V, Sumycin)

    Chlamydia is caused by *Chlamydia trachomatis,* a gram-negative coccus. Drugs used to treat chlamydia infections include:

      demeclocycline (Declomycin)
      doxycycline (Vibramycin)
      erythromycin (E.E.S., E-Mycin, Eryc, Ilotycin)
      methacycline (Rondomycin)
      minocycline (Minocin)
      tetracycline (Achromycin V, Sumycin)

    Herpes simplex virus, type 2, genital lesions may be treated with topical acyclovir (Zovirax) or the lesions may be injected intradermally with these drugs.

      interferon alfa-2b (Intron A)
      interferon alfa-n3 (Alferon N)

    Women with sexually transmitted diseases can transmit them to their newborn infants in utero or via the infected birth canal. Systemic infections from gonorrhea or syphilis are treated as above. In addition, most states either recommend or require the use of a topical anti-infective agent to be applied to the eyes of newborn infants to prevent infection and possible blindness caused by gonorrhea and *Chlamydia.* Topical solutions and ointments specially prepared for ophthalmic use to prevent gonorrhea include:

      silver nitrate
      erythromycin (Ilotycin)
      tetracycline (Achromycin)

Silver nitrate is ineffective in preventing eye infections due to *Chlamydia.* Instead, erythromycin or tetracycline is applied topically.

Miscellaneous Drugs

bromocriptine (Parlodel) This drug activates dopamine receptors in the brain which in turn release a substance which inhibits the production of prolactin. Prolactin is normally secreted by the pituitary gland to stimulate milk production during pregnancy and lactation. Bromocriptine (Parlodel) inhibits milk production and breast engorgement in mothers who choose not to breast feed and may also be used for women who have had stillborn infants or abortions.

DID YOU KNOW? Bromocriptine (Parlodel) is also used to treat Parkinson disease. By activating dopamine receptors, this drug helps to make up for the lack of natural dopamine in the brain which causes parkinsonian symptoms.

Enovid A combination of estrogen and progesterone used to treat hypermenorrhea.

Hyskon This fluid is used intraoperatively to distend the uterine cavity and facilitate visualization with the hysteroscope.

magnesium sulfate Given I.V., this drug is used to prevent and control the seizures associated with preeclampsia and eclampsia.

DID YOU KNOW? Magnesium sulfate is also manufactured in a nonsterile crystalline form which is mixed with water and drunk as a laxative. Its name is Epsom salt.

MICRhoGAM See *RhoGAM*.

RhoGAM Given I.M., this immunoglobulin drug is used to suppress the immune response in Rh negative women who have just delivered an Rh positive baby (or had an abortion, miscarriage, or amniocentesis). During pregnancy, some of the baby's Rh positive red blood cells enter the mother's bloodstream. The Rh negative mother then develops antibodies against these Rh positive red blood cells. This does not affect the first infant while it is in the womb, but the red blood cells of Rh positive babies in subsequent pregnancies will be attacked by the maternal antibodies. These babies can develop hemolytic disease of the newborn. RhoGAM is given only to Rh negative mothers whose babies, when blood typing is performed after birth, are Rh positive. In cases where the baby's blood type cannot be determined (such as during amniocentesis), RhoGAM is given prophylactically. RhoGAM is never given to the infant. For women who have a miscarriage or abortion prior to 12 weeks of gestation, MICRhoGAM (a micro-dose of the immunoglobulin in RhoGAM) is given.

24

Neurological Drugs

Various disease conditions of the central nervous system benefit from pharmacologic therapy. These include epilepsy, Parkinson disease, insomnia, and attention deficit disorder.

Drugs for Epilepsy

An epileptic seizure originates in the brain when a group of neurons begin to spontaneously send out impulses in an abnormal, uncontrolled way. These impulses

HISTORICAL NOTE: Efforts to control epilepsy were largely in vain for centuries. The cause was attributed to supernatural forces, poison, etc. The treatment could involve trephining (boring a hole in the skull), prayers, or herbal remedies. Phenobarbital (Luminal), the first drug effective for epilepsy (tonic-clonic seizures only) was introduced in 1912.

"In 1923, young Tracy Putnam became a resident in neurology. . . . He became intrigued with the possibility that epilepsy might be caused by a chemical abnormality in the brain. He noted, for example, that patients who 'rebreathed' their own carbon dioxide by putting a bag over their heads got some relief. He asked himself, 'Might an institution for the treatment of epilepsy be established adjacent to a brewery, and the content of carbon dioxide in the atmosphere metered so as to be tolerable and yet sufficient to prevent attacks?'"

Putnam abandoned this idea and instead began searching for drugs which might be effective for epilepsy. "'I combed the catalog,' Putnam later wrote, 'for suitable compounds that were not obviously poisonous.' He was looking for drugs in particular containing a benzene ring, because among the barbitals, only phenobarbital, which also had a benzene ring, possessed the ability to suppress epilepsy. 'Parke-Davis . . . wrote back to me that it had on hand samples of nineteen different compounds analogous to phenobarbital and that I was welcome to them.'" (Edward Shorter, Ph.D., *The Health Century* [New York: Doubleday, 1987], pp. 110-111.)

Of the nineteen in the shipment, all were inactive and ineffective against epilepsy except one—phenytoin (Dilantin), which was introduced in 1938 and is the drug of choice for treating tonic-clonic seizures.

are spread from neuron to neuron by neurotransmitter hormones. Symptoms of epilepsy range from barely noticeable staring or a lack of attention to a full tonic-clonic seizure with muscle jerking, tongue biting, and incontinence. The extent of the symptoms depends on the number and location of the affected neurons. Each type of epilepsy displays a specific EEG pattern during a seizure. The choice of drug therapy is dependent upon proper classification of the type of seizure based on clinical symptoms and the EEG pattern. There are four common types of seizures: tonic-clonic (formerly known as grand mal), absence (formerly known as petit mal), complex partial (formerly known as psychomotor), and simple partial (formerly known as focal motor).

There is no one drug which has therapeutic effects against all types of seizures. Some drugs which are effective for controlling one type of seizure may actually provoke another type of seizure.

Barbiturates are a class of sedative drugs, some of which possess an anticonvulsant action. Barbiturates are Schedule III and IV drugs which act to inhibit conduction of nerve impulses to the cortex of the brain, and to depress motor areas of the brain. Barbiturates used to treat seizures include:

    mephobarbital (Mebaral)
    metharbital (Gemonil)
    phenobarbital (Luminal)

Hydantoins are a class of drugs which act on cell membranes of neurons in the cortex of the brain. These drugs affect the flow of sodium in and out of the cell thereby preventing it from depolarizing and repolarizing (i.e., sending out an impulse) rapidly and repeatedly. Hydantoins used to treat seizures include:

    ethotoin (Peganone)
    mephenytoin (Mesantoin)
    phenytoin (Dilantin)

Succinimides are a class of drugs which act to depress the cortex and raise the seizure threshold. They include:

    ethosuximide (Zarontin)
    methsuximide (Celontin)
    phensuximide (Milontin)

Drugs used to treat tonic-clonic seizures include:

    carbamazepine (Tegretol)
    ethotoin (Peganone)
    mephenytoin (Mesantoin)
    mephobarbital (Mebaral)—a Schedule III barbiturate
    metharbital (Gemonil)—a Schedule III barbiturate
    phenobarbital (Luminal)—a Schedule IV barbiturate
    phenytoin (Dilantin)
    primidone (Mysoline)

Note: Phenytoin (Dilantin) is the drug of choice for treating adults with tonic-clonic seizures, while phenobarbital (Luminal) is the drug of choice for treating children.

Drugs used to treat absence seizures include:
   acetazolamide (Diamox)
   clonazepam (Klonopin)
   ethosuximide (Zarontin)
   mephobarbital (Mebaral)—a Schedule III barbiturate
   metharbital (Gemonil)—a Schedule III barbiturate
   methsuximide (Celontin)
   paramethadione (Paradione)
   phensuximide (Milontin)
   primidone (Mysoline)
   trimethadione (Tridione)
   valproic acid (Depakene, Depakote)
Note: Ethosuximide (Zarontin) is the drug of choice for treating absence seizures.
   Drugs used to treat complex partial seizures include:
   carbamazepine (Tegretol)
   clorazepate (Tranxene)
   ethotoin (Peganone)
   mephenytoin (Mesantoin)
   phenacemide (Phenurone)
   phenytoin (Dilantin)
   primidone (Mysoline)
Drugs used to treat simple partial seizures include:
   clorazepate (Tranxene)
   mephenytoin (Mesantoin)
   phenobarbital (Luminal)
   primidone (Mysoline)

Drugs to Treat Parkinson Disease

The symptoms of Parkinson disease were first described in 1817 by the English physician James Parkinson. Parkinson disease is a chronic, degenerative condition affecting the brain. Its early symptoms, first appearing usually in adults of late middle age, include muscle rigidity, tremors, and a slowing of voluntary movements. Parkinson disease follows a progressively downhill clinical course. Later symptoms include a mask-like facial expression and drooling from rigidity of the facial muscles, resting tremor, and loss of ability to ambulate.

The symptoms of Parkinson disease may be attributed to a disturbance in the balance of dopamine and acetylcholine, two neurotransmitters in the brain. These two substances normally exert opposing, balancing effects. It is a lack of dopamine in the brain that upsets this delicate balance leading to the symptoms of Parkinson disease.

Drug therapy for Parkinson disease is divided into two main categories: drugs which increase or enhance the action of dopamine in the brain, and drugs which inhibit the action of acetylcholine. All of these drugs act to restore the natural balance between dopamine and acetylcholine.

IN DEPTH: Direct attempts to replenish the diminished supply of dopamine in the brain were unsuccessful because dopamine given orally and circulating in the blood cannot cross the blood-brain barrier. It was discovered, however, that the metabolic precursor of dopamine, levodopa, could not only penetrate the blood-brain barrier but could actually increase brain levels of dopamine. Once in the brain, levodopa (or L-dopa) is converted into dopamine by the action of the enzyme dopa decarboxylase. Unfortunately, this same enzyme is also present in the bloodstream.

After oral administration of levodopa, this enzyme begins immediately to change levodopa in the bloodstream into dopamine which cannot cross the blood-brain barrier. This results in two problems: (1) A very large oral dose of levodopa must be given because a substantial amount (97-99%) of the levodopa in the blood is converted into dopamine by this enzyme; thus, its therapeutic effect is lost. (2) The extra dopamine in the bloodstream causes side effects which are undesirable.

To avoid both of these problems, levodopa is given orally along with another drug, carbidopa. Carbidopa inhibits the enzyme dopa decarboxylase to allow a higher circulating level of levodopa to cross the blood-brain barrier. The use of carbidopa allows the dose of levodopa to be decreased by 75%. Fortunately, oral carbidopa cannot cross the blood-brain barrier to inhibit the enzyme dopa decarboxylase in the brain where it is needed to change levodopa into dopamine.

Drugs which increase the amount of dopamine, enhance its action in the brain, or directly stimulate dopamine receptors include:

> amantadine (Symmetrel)
> bromocriptine (Parlodel)
> carbidopa (Lodosyn)
> levodopa (L-dopa, Larodopa)
> pergolide mesylate (Permax)
> selegiline (Eldepryl)

DID YOU KNOW? Amantadine (Symmetrel) was originally used as an antiviral agent to prevent the Asian flu. It was given for this reason to a patient at Harvard Medical School who had also had Parkinson disease. By coincidence, it was noted that his Parkinson disease improved. Today, amantadine (Symmetrel) is also given to high-risk patients to prevent influenza A virus infections.

DID YOU KNOW? Bromocriptine (Parlodel) is also given to suppress lactation in mothers who do not wish to breast-feed their babies after delivery (or following a miscarriage or abortion). Bromocriptine activates dopamine receptors which in turn release a substance that inhibits the production of prolactin, the hormone which stimulates milk production.

Drugs which inhibit the action of acetylcholine in the brain include:
    benztropine mesylate (Cogentin)
    biperiden (Akineton)
    ethopropazine (Parsidol)
    procyclidine (Kemadrin)
    trihexyphenidyl (Artane)
Combination drugs for Parkinson disease include:
    Sinemet-10/100 (mg of carbidopa/mg of levodopa)
    Sinemet-25/100
    Sinemet-25/250
None of the drugs prescribed for Parkinson disease can cure it. In fact, over time tolerance can develop to their therapeutic effects. Larger drug doses are then required to maintain control of parkinsonian symptoms; however, these also produce more side effects. When doses can no longer be increased or when side effects become intolerable, the physician will gradually withdraw all medication, placing the patient on a **"drug holiday"** for a few days. When drug therapy is again initiated, the patient will respond to lower doses of antiparkinsonian drugs.

Drugs used to treat seizures associated with preeclampsia/eclampsia are discussed in Chapter 23.

Drugs used to treat migraine headaches are discussed in Chapter 26.

Drugs for Insomnia

Drugs which are used to induce sleep are termed *hypnotics* after *hypnos,* the Greek word for sleep. **Hypnotics** may be either nonbarbiturates which carry a low risk of addiction, or **barbiturates** (Schedule II or III drugs) which are more addictive and are the second choice for treating insomnia.

Nonbarbiturate hypnotics. Nonbarbiturate hypnotics nonselectively depress central nervous system functions and promote sedation and sleep. These drugs have a low incidence of addiction and are greatly preferred over barbiturates for the treatment of simple insomnia. These drugs are, for the most part, Schedule IV. Nonbarbiturate hypnotics include:
    chloral hydrate (Noctec)
    estazolam (ProSom)—an investigational drug
    ethchlorvynol (Placidyl)
    ethinamate (Valmid)
    flurazepam (Dalmane)

glutethimide (Doriden)
methyprylon (Noludar)
quazepam (Doral)
temazepam (Restoril)
triazolam (Halcion)

Flurazepam (Dalmane) is the most common hypnotic prescribed for insomnia.

Note: The ending *-azepam* is common to generic benzodiazepines, some of which are used as hypnotics. Other benzodiazepines are commonly used as minor tranquilizers for anxiety.

Nonbarbiturate over-the-counter sleep aids (such as Sominex, Nytol, and Unisom) commonly contain the antihistamine diphenhydramine (Benadryl). These sleep aids use the antihistamine's side effect of drowsiness as the therapeutic effect to treat insomnia. They are not schedule drugs.

Barbiturate hypnotics. Some barbiturates, as mentioned previously, are useful in preventing epileptic seizures. Others have no anticonvulsant activity and are used to treat insomnia. They produce a general depressing action on the central nervous system and sedation. However, barbiturate hypnotics are Schedule II and III drugs and, because of their greater ability to cause addiction, are not preferred over the nonbarbiturate hypnotics. Barbiturate hypnotics include:

aprobarbital (Alurate)
butabarbital (Butisol)
pentobarbital (Nembutal)
secobarbital (Seconal)
talbutal (Lotusate)

Note: The ending *-barbital* is common to many generic barbiturates.

Drugs for Attention Deficit Disorder

Hyperactive children exhibit extreme symptoms of restlessness, short attention span, distractibility, emotional lability, and impulsive or disruptive behavior. This complex of symptoms has been known as minimal brain dysfunction and is now termed attention deficit disorder (ADD). The cause of ADD may be brain damage at birth, genetic factors, or other abnormalities. It is five times more common in boys than in girls. Most children outgrow the symptoms of ADD in late childhood. Drugs used to treat ADD are amphetamines and other related CNS-stimulating drugs. They have a paradoxical reverse effect in children in that they do not overstimulate behavior but actually reduce impulse behavior and increase the attention span. Drug therapy for ADD is accompanied by psychological counseling as well as special education intervention. Drugs for ADD include:

amphetamine—a Schedule II drug
dextroamphetamine (Dexedrine)—a Schedule II drug
methamphetamine (Desoxyn)—a Schedule II drug
methylphenidate (Ritalin)
pemoline (Cylert)
Obetrol-20 (amphetamine and dextroamphetamine)

DID YOU KNOW? Amphetamine was synthesized in the late 1920s. It became a drug of abuse during World War II to help maintain alertness and avoid battle fatigue. During the 1960s, methamphetamine (''speed'') became a popular drug of abuse. In 1972, amphetamines were classified as Schedule II drugs with a high potential for abuse.

Miscellaneous Drugs

chlordiazepoxide (Librium)   A benzodiazepine antianxiety drug with a special application for the prevention of seizures during alcoholic detoxification.

diazepam (Valium)   A benzodiazepine antianxiety drug with a special application for treating the constant, intractable seizures of status epilepticus.

mannitol (Osmitrol)   A diuretic used to relieve cerebral edema and decrease intracranial pressure.

paraldehyde   A sedative/hypnotic used to decrease agitation and promote sedation and sleep in patients undergoing alcohol withdrawal.

tacrine (Cognex)   An investigational anticholinergic drug which inhibits the action of acetylcholine in the brain and helps to improve memory function in patients with Alzheimer disease.

Tuinal   A combination of amobarbital and secobarbital for sedation or insomnia.

REVIEW QUESTIONS

1. Zarontin is the drug of choice for tonic-clonic seizures. True or False?
2. Why is levodopa administered with carbidopa for patients with Parkinson disease?
3. What two very distinct and different medical uses does the drug bromocriptine (Parlodel) have?
4. Why is a central nervous system stimulant given to hyperactive children with attention deficit disorder?

SPELLING TIPS

- phenytoin (The drug is easily misspelled because the *y* is not usually pronounced.)

25

Psychiatric Drugs

The term *mental illness* encompasses a variety of emotional disorders which involve abnormalities of personality, mood, or behavior. It is estimated that nearly 50% of all hospital admissions are in some way related to a mental health problem such as anxiety, depression, suicide, postpartum depression, psychosis, psychosomatic illness, senility, child abuse, drug addiction, or alcoholism.

HISTORICAL NOTE: During the 1800s, the treatment for mental illness could include the use of the drugs digitalis, ipecac, alcohol, or opium. In 1903 barbiturates were synthesized and used effectively as sedative drugs for agitated mentally ill patients. They have largely been replaced by newer drugs. Before World War II, schizophrenic patients were treated in several ways. They could be exposed to malaria to produce a high fever and delirium, they could be injected with enough insulin to cause convulsions and coma, or they could be given electroshock therapy. Amphetamines were used to alleviate depression.

Beginning in the early 1950s, there were advances made in the treatment of mental illness with the introduction of new drugs to treat neurosis, psychosis, and depression.

The broad category of mental illnesses can be divided into many subcategories, of which we will consider only neurosis, psychosis, and affective disorders and their respective drug therapies.

Drugs for Neurosis

The symptoms of neurosis include anxiety, anxiousness, and tension—all at a more intense level than normal—and a feeling of apprehension with vague, unsubstantiated fears. The neurotic patient, however, never experiences any loss of touch with reality.

The treatment of neurosis involves the use of **antianxiety drugs,** also known as **anxiolytic agents** or minor tranquilizers. The term **minor tranquilizer** is somewhat of a misnomer in that it carries the connotation that this class of drugs is somehow less effective in treating symptoms than the major tranquilizers (used to treat psychosis) or that the minor tranquilizers are only major tranquilizers given at a lower dose. In fact, minor tranquilizers are completely unrelated chemically to major tranquilizers. They are extremely effective drugs of great importance with specific therapeutic action in treating neurosis.

HISTORICAL NOTE: In 1945 researchers were looking for a new antibiotic to use against bacteria that were already becoming resistant to penicillin. One drug tested was found to produce muscle relaxation and exert a calming effect in animals. From this parent molecule, the first minor tranquilizer was developed in 1955 and marketed as meprobamate (Equanil, Miltown).

In 1955 a researcher at Hoffmann-La Roche laboratories had been searching for a compound for making commercial dye, but the chemicals he developed were not useful as dyes. A year and a half of research yielded no usable products. As he was doing his final cleaning up of the project, he noted a single sample which he had forgotten to send for testing. He notes, ''We were under great pressure by this time because my boss told us to stop these foolish things and go back to more useful work. I submitted it [the sample] for animal testing. . . . I thought myself that it was just to finish up.'' (Edward Shorter, Ph.D., *The Health Century* [New York: Doubleday, 1987], p. 127.)

That last sample which was nearly forgotten turned out to be chlordiazepoxide (Librium), which was released for sale in 1960, the first of the benzodiazepine class of minor tranquilizers that would come to dominate the treatment of neurosis.

The same researcher continued to work with the basic molecular structure of chlordiazepoxide (Librium), and in 1959, even before marketing of Librium had begun, he had synthesized the new drug diazepam (Valium). (See Fig. 25-1.) The trade name *Valium* is derived from the Latin word *valere* which means *to be healthy*. In 1970 Valium became the number one prescription drug in the United States. Even ten years later, Hoffman-La Roche was still manufacturing 30 million Valium tablets every day.

Benzodiazepines. The benzodiazepines are by far the most commonly prescribed drugs for the treatment of anxiety and neurosis. They bind to several specific types of receptor sites in the brain to provide sedation and affect thought processes; they affect emotional behavior by their action in the limbic area of the brain; and in the spinal cord they decrease the muscle tension that comes with anxiety. All of the benzodiazepines are Schedule IV drugs and include:

     alprazolam (Xanax)
     chlordiazepoxide (Librium)
     clorazepate (Tranxene)
     clobazam (Frisium)—an investigational drug
     diazepam (Valium)
     halazepam (Paxipam)
     lorazepam (Ativan)

oxazepam (Serax)

prazepam (Centrax)

Note: The ending -*azepam* is common to generic benzodiazepine drugs used to treat anxiety/neurosis.

Other drugs used to treat neurosis include:

buspirone (BuSpar)

chlormezanone (Trancopal)

doxepin (Adapin, Sinequan)

meprobamate (Equanil, Miltown, Meprospan)—a Schedule IV drug

Librium   Valium

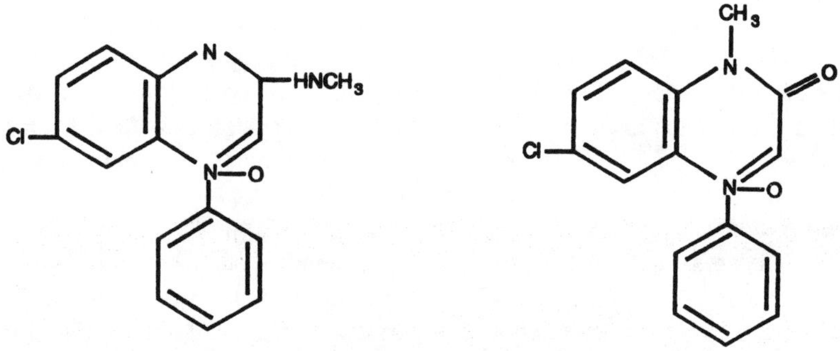

FIGURE 25-1

The similar chemical structures of chlordiazepoxide (Librium) and diazepam (Valium), the first two benzodiazepine minor tranquilizers.

Drugs Used to Treat Psychosis

The symptoms of psychosis include a loss of touch with reality with resulting illusions, delusions, and hallucinations. Psychotic symptomatology may, in part, be based on an overactivity of the neurotransmitter dopamine in the brain either from overproduction of dopamine or from hypersensitivity of dopamine receptors.

The treatment of psychosis involves the use of **antipsychotic drugs**, which are also known as **major tranquilizers** or **neuroleptics**. These drugs block dopamine receptors in many areas of the brain including the limbic system which controls emotions. Antipsychotic drugs decrease hostility, agitation, and paranoia without causing confusion or sedation. None of the antipsychotic drugs are addictive; they are not schedule drugs.

Phenothiazine drugs for psychosis include:

acetophenazine (Tindal)

chlorpromazine (Thorazine)

fluphenazine (Prolixin)

mesoridazine (Serentil)

perphenazine (Trilafon)

promazine (Sparine)

HISTORICAL NOTE: Prior to the introduction of modern antipsychotic drugs, barbiturates were used to sedate agitated psychotic patients. These drugs have been replaced by the phenothiazine group of drugs which are just as effective but produce no sedation. Phenothiazine was the original parent drug for this group of antipsychotic agents. It was first manufactured in 1883 and was used as a wormer for livestock. Some minor changes in its chemical structure resulted in the creation of chlorpromazine (Thorazine), the first of the modern antipsychotic drugs and still one of the most widely used.

thioridazine (Mellaril)
trifluoperazine (Stelazine)
triflupromazine (Vesprin)
Note: The ending -*azine* is common to generic phenothiazine antipsychotic drugs.
Other antipsychotic drugs which are not of the phenothiazine group include:
chlorprothixene (Taractan)
haloperidol (Haldol)
loxapine (Loxitane)
molindone (Moban)
thiothixene (Navane)

Drugs Used to Treat Affective Disorders

The term *affect* refers to an emotional feeling or mood expressed by a patient's outward appearance. Affective disorders center on two major emotions: **depression** and **mania**. The depressed patient experiences insomnia, crying, lack of pleasure in any activity, loss of appetite, suicidal feelings, and feelings of helplessness,

HISTORICAL NOTE: Originally, amphetamines were used to treat depression by stimulating the central nervous system and masking the patient's depressive symptoms. Amphetamines have a high potential for abuse and do not correct the underlying chemical imbalance causing depression; therefore, they are no longer used to treat depression.

In 1951, while evaluating a drug for its effectiveness in treating tuberculosis, researchers noted that even seriously ill and dying patients developed a happy, optimistic attitude despite the lack of clinical improvement in their tuberculosis. This drug was identified as a monoamine oxidase (MAO) inhibitor, and it formed the basis for the first class of drugs used to treat depression—MAO inhibitors.

In 1958 a drug being tested as an antipsychotic showed significant antidepressant effects. That drug was imipramine (Tofranil) and it was the first of the tricyclic antidepressant drugs, so named for their characteristic three-ring structure. (See Fig. 25-3.) In 1981 the tetracyclic antidepressant class was introduced with maprotiline (Ludiomil).

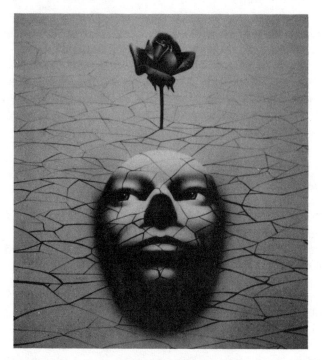

FIGURE 25-2
Depression—"a disease that affects millions of people throughout the world, the sufferers of which can truly be called the wretched of the earth." This illustration for the tetracyclic antidepressant maprotiline (Ludiomil) is reprinted here, courtesy of Ciba Pharmaceutical.

hopelessness, and worthlessness. Depression results from decreased levels of the neurotransmitters norepinephrine and serotonin in the brain. The treatment for depression involves the use of **antidepressant drugs.**

Antidepressants, or **mood-elevating drugs,** not only alleviate the symptoms of depression, they also increase mental alertness, normalize sleep patterns, help restore appetite, and decrease suicidal ideation. There are three main categories of antidepressant drugs: monoamine oxidase (MAO) inhibitors, tricyclic antidepressants, and tetracyclic antidepressants.

Monoamine oxidase (MAO) inhibitors for depression. This older group of antidepressants prevents the enzyme monoamine oxidase (MAO) from breaking down the neurotransmitter norepinephrine in the brain. MAO inhibitor drugs are used infrequently due to the possibility of severe side effects.

MAO inhibitors used to treat depression include:
isocarboxazid (Marplan)
phenelzine (Nardil)
tranylcypromine (Parnate)

IN DEPTH: The enzyme monoamine oxidase normally breaks down norepinephrine (in the brain) as well as tyramine (in the intestine) obtained from
the diet. Because the enzyme is blocked when a person takes an MAO inhibitor,
tyramine is not metabolized properly. Tyramine in the diet is absorbed intact
directly into the bloodstream. The excess tyramine in the blood stimulates the
release of stored norepinephrine in large quantities, and this results in violent
headaches, severe hypertension, and possible stroke. This can occur quickly
if a patient taking MAO inhibitors for depression ingests food which contains
high levels of tyramine. These foods include aged cheese, wine, beer, chicken
liver, bananas, bologna, salami, sausage, avocados, chocolate, and coffee.
Because of these dietary restrictions, these drugs are only occasionally used
to treat depression that fails to respond to other antidepressant drugs.

Tricyclic antidepressant drugs. The tricyclic antidepressants prolong the action of norepinephrine in the brain and correct its low levels which cause depression. The tricyclics are so named because of the triple-ring configuration of their
chemical structure. (See Fig. 25-3.)

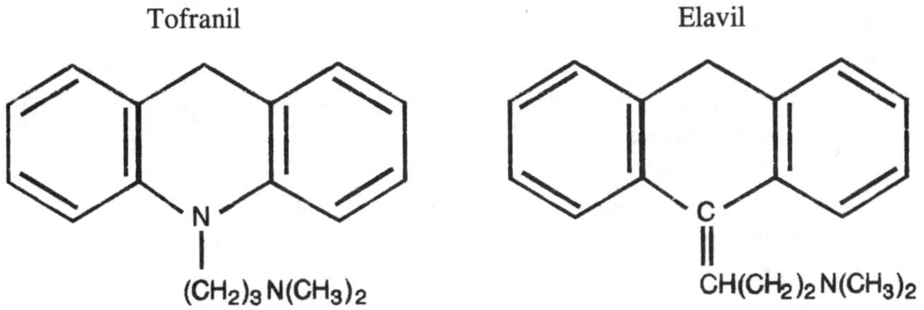

Tofranil

Elavil

$(CH_2)_3 N(CH_3)_2$

$CH(CH_2)_2 N(CH_3)_2$

FIGURE 25-3
Chemical structure of the tricyclic antidepressants imipramine (Tofranil) and amitriptyline
(Elavil), showing the three-ring structure from which they derive their name.

The tricyclic antidepressants include:
    amitriptyline (Elavil, Endep)
    amoxapine (Asendin)
    desipramine (Norpramin)
    dothiepin (Prothiaden)—an investigational drug
    doxepin (Adapin, Sinequan)
    imipramine (Tofranil)
    nortriptyline (Aventyl, Pamelor)
    protriptyline (Vivactil)
    trimipramine (Surmontil)

Note: The endings *-triptyline* and *-ipramine* are common to many tricyclic antidepressants.

Tetracyclic antidepressant drugs. Although slightly different in chemical structure, tetracyclic antidepressants have the same therapeutic effect as the tricyclic antidepressants described above. At the present time, there is only one drug on the market in this class of antidepressants.

maprotiline (Ludiomil)

Other antidepressant drugs which act to inhibit the uptake of serotonin in the brain so as to correct its low levels include:

bupropion (Wellbutrin)
fluoxetine (Prozac)
trazodone (Desyrel)

Lithium. The second emotion of affective disorders is that of **mania,** which is associated with increased levels of norepinephrine in the brain. Mania coupled with depression is known as manic-depressive disorder or bipolar disorder because the patient's mood swings between two opposite poles of emotion.

Lithium (Eskalith, Lithobid, Lithotabs) is used exclusively to treat the symptoms of manic-depressive illness. Lithium inhibits the continued action of norepinephrine to suppress manic symptoms caused by too much norepinephrine, and it increases the action of serotonin to correct the depression caused by low levels of serotonin. Lithium lessens the severity of mood swings from depression to mania and decreases the frequency with which these cycles occur.

Combination Drugs for Treating Mental Illness

Deprol (an antianxiety drug and an antidepressant)
Equagesic (an antianxiety drug and aspirin)
Etrafon (an antipsychotic and an antidepressant)
Librax (an antianxiety drug with a GI antispasmodic drug)
Limbitrol DS (an antianxiety drug and an antidepressant)
Triavil (an antipsychotic and an antidepressant)

Miscellaneous Drugs

clomipramine (Anafranil)   This antidepressant is used specifically to treat patients with obsessive-compulsive behavior disorders; it is the only drug on the market for this problem.

clozapine (Clozaril)   An antipsychotic drug used specifically for schizophrenic patients who fail to respond to other antipsychotic drugs.

disulfiram (Antabuse)   Given to alcoholics to prevent them from consuming alcohol, this drug inhibits an enzyme which normally metabolizes acetaldehyde (one of the breakdown products of alcohol) in the bloodstream. If the patient drinks alcohol while taking disulfiram, the alcohol is oxidized to acetaldehyde but cannot be metabolized further. Acetaldehyde levels become greatly increased, causing symptoms of flushing, headache, dizziness, nausea, and possibly even severe hypotension and arrhythmias. These adverse reactions are supposed to keep alcoholic patients from taking a drink. However, patients cannot be placed on disulfiram without first giving consent and being thoroughly forewarned of the dangerous complications of alcohol consumption. Compliance with this drug regimen is strictly voluntary. Patients must also be warned to avoid cough syrups, mouthwashes, and aftershaves containing alcohol.

Hydergine. Used to treat Alzheimer disease, this drug increases brain metabolism and blood flow.

HISTORICAL NOTE: Disulfiram (Antabuse) was originally used in the commercial production of rubber. In 1948 two Danish researchers began testing this drug for its possible effectiveness in treating intestinal worms. To study its safety in humans, they both took the drug. When each became ill after consuming alcohol, they concluded that the alcohol-disulfiram combination had produced the reaction. Antabuse was first prescribed for the prevention of alcoholism that same year.

REVIEW QUESTIONS

1. Minor tranquilizers are the same drugs as major tranquilizers but are given at a lower dosage. True or False?
2. Give three names assigned to all of the drugs used to treat psychosis.
3. The terms *tricyclic* and *tetracyclic* bring to mind what class of drugs?
4. Name the only drug that is available to treat each of these conditions.
   - alcoholism (to prevent drinking)   drug: _____
   - manic-depressive disorder   drug: _____
   - obsessive-compulsive behavior   drug: _____

SPELLING TIPS

- Asendin (The name implies helping patients ascend from the depths of depression, but the c in *ascend* has been deleted in *Asendin*.)
- Antabuse (Not *Antiabuse*; there is no *i*.)

26

Analgesic Drugs

Drugs for pain can be divided into three large categories: narcotic, non-narcotic, and nonsteroidal anti-inflammatory drugs (NSAIDs).

The ideal analgesic drug would provide maximum pain relief, produce no side effects, and cause no dependence or addiction. Unfortunately, the ideal analgesic drug does not exist. Drugs which effectively relieve severe pain are usually addictive (narcotics), while non-narcotic and NSAIDs are effective only for mild to moderately severe pain.

Narcotic Analgesics

The term *narcotic* is derived from the Greek word *narke* which means *numbness*. Narcotic drugs relieve pain by binding with opiate receptor sites in the brain to block pain impulses to the brain from ascending neural pathways. Natural opiate-like substances in the body (such as **endorphins**) normally occupy these receptors and produce a natural type of pain relief. There are several different types of opiate receptors which account for the stronger addicting quality of some narcotic drugs as compared to others and their different classifications as schedule drugs. The existence of different opiate receptors also accounts for the different kinds of side effects seen with various narcotic drugs.

Common side effects of narcotics include constipation, respiratory depression, sedation, and euphoria. It is the presence of significant euphoria which causes some narcotic drugs to be more psychologically addicting than others. One common narcotic side effect, suppression of the cough center (antitussive effect), is used as a therapeutic effect by including certain narcotic drugs in cough syrups (example: Hycodan). See Chapter 19, page 99. For narcotic drugs which use the side effect of constipation as a therapeutic effect to treat diarrhea, see Chapter 13, page 64.

Narcotic drugs may be directly derived from opium or may be synthetically manufactured.

Narcotic drugs are used to treat moderate to severe pain; provide preoperative and postoperative pain relief, sedation, and a feeling of well-being (euphoria); and to maintain general anesthesia (see Chapter 31, page 160).

Narcotic drugs given by mouth or by injection for pain control include:

buprenorphine (Buprenex)	Schedule V drug
butorphanol (Stadol)	Not a schedule drug

codeine	Schedule II drug
dezocine (Dalgan)	Not a schedule drug
hydromorphone (Dilaudid)	Schedule II drug
levorphanol (Levo-Dromoran)	Schedule II drug
meperidine (Demerol)	Schedule II drug
methadone (Dolophine)	Schedule II drug
morphine sulfate (Duramorph, MS Contin)	Schedule II drug
nalbuphine (Nubain)	Not a schedule drug
opium (Pantopon)	Schedule III drug
oxycodone (Roxicodone)	Schedule II drug
oxymorphone (Numorphan)	Schedule II drug
pentazocine (Talwin)	Schedule IV drug
propoxyphene (Darvon)	Schedule IV drug

DID YOU KNOW? Opium is obtained from the dried seeds of the poppy. Morphine was first isolated from opium in 1815. Morphine was named for the Greek god of dreams, Morpheus, who was the son of Hypnos, the Greek god of sleep. Morphine was used extensively during the Civil War, resulting in a very high rate of addiction among veterans. Heroin, a semisynthetic narcotic, was introduced in 1898 as a nonaddicting substitute for morphine. It proved to be more addicting and, at the present time, is classified as a Schedule I drug with no medical uses. In 1939 meperidine (Demerol), the first synthetic narcotic drug, was introduced.

Non-narcotic Analgesics

Non-narcotic analgesics are used to treat mild to moderate pain associated with many disease conditions. These drugs include salicylates and acetaminophen. Non-narcotic analgesics are the first step in pain control and have the advantage over narcotic analgesics by being nonaddicting and less expensive. In fact, most non-narcotic analgesics are available over-the-counter unless they are offered in combination with a narcotic drug. However, non-narcotic analgesics are not as effective as narcotics for the relief of sharp or severe pain.

Salicylates

Salicylate is a general term which includes aspirin and other chemically related compounds.

DID YOU KNOW? Aspirin was first introduced in 1899, although for many years previously it was used for pain relief in its natural form from willow bark. Aspirin is also known as acetylsalicylic acid (abbreviated ASA) from the Latin word *salix*, meaning *willow*.

Aspirin. Aspirin has four distinct therapeutic actions:
- Analgesic. It provides relief of pain by inhibiting the release of prostaglandins from damaged tissue.
- Anti-inflammatory. It decreases inflammation by inhibiting the release of prostaglandins from damaged tissue.
- Antipyretic. It reduces fever by acting on the hypothalamus to cause general vasodilation and sweating which increases heat loss from the skin.
- Anticoagulant. It prolongs the clotting time by inhibiting thromboxane which normally causes platelets to aggregate.

Aspirin is marketed under the following trade names:

A.S.A. Enseals
Ascriptin A/D
Bayer Aspirin
Bufferin
Cama
Easprin
Ecotrin

Because salicylic acid is irritating to the stomach, long-term therapy may produce stomach ulcers. To reduce this irritation, aspirin may be manufactured as an enteric-coated tablet (Ecotrin), which will dissolve only in the higher pH environment of the duodenum. Aspirin may also be combined with antacids such as magnesium or aluminum to protect the stomach (Ascriptin A/D, Bufferin, Cama).

Aspirin has long been a basic treatment for rheumatoid arthritis, treating both the pain and inflammation. Another newer use for aspirin has been as an anticoagulant for patients who have had a myocardial infarction. One tablet of aspirin daily has been shown to significantly decrease the incidence of a second heart attack. Aspirin is also used prophylactically as an anticoagulant in patients with a history of transient ischemic attacks (small, recurring strokes).

Note: In the past few years, the use of aspirin to treat the aches and pains of a viral illness has been linked to the occurrence of **Reye syndrome** in young children. Reye syndrome can cause liver damage due to increased serum levels of ammonia, and can cause encephalitis. Therefore, the symptomatic treatment of colds, flu, and chickenpox with aspirin is no longer recommended for children.

Other salicylates. Other salicylate drugs with therapeutic actions similar to aspirin include:

Arthropan
diflunisal (Dolobid)
Trilisate

Acetaminophen

Acetaminophen has two distinct therapeutic actions:
- Analgesic. The mechanism by which it relieves pain is unclear.
- Antipyretic. It reduces fever by acting on the hypothalamus to cause vasodilation and sweating which increase heat loss from the skin.

> DID YOU KNOW? The antipyretic action of acetaminophen was discovered in 1887 when it was given to a patient with intestinal parasites and his fever was reduced. However, the use of acetaminophen did not become widespread until it was introduced under the trade name Tylenol in 1955.

Acetaminophen has no anti-inflammatory properties and is not effective in treating rheumatoid arthritis. It also has no anticoagulant effect and therefore is not given to prevent second heart attacks or transient ischemic attacks.

Acetaminophen is marketed under the following trade names:

Anacin-3
Datril
Liquiprin
Panadol
Tempra
Tylenol

Combination Non-Narcotic Analgesic Drugs

The following drugs contain aspirin and/or acetaminophen for pain relief and caffeine as a stimulant and vasoconstrictor.

Anacin (aspirin and caffeine)
Excedrin (aspirin, acetaminophen, and caffeine)
Synalgos (aspirin and caffeine)
Trigesic (aspirin, acetaminophen, and caffeine)
Vanquish (aspirin, acetaminophen, and caffeine)

Combination Narcotic and Non-Narcotic Drugs

Narcotic and non-narcotic drugs are often given in combination with each other for two reasons: (1) The non-narcotic drug provides a foundation of pain relief upon which the narcotic drug can build; therefore, less narcotic is needed. (2) This combination of drugs acts against the two components of pain—pain which results from actual stimulation of nerve endings, and pain which is initiated and heightened by anxiety. Drugs which combine narcotic and non-narcotic pain relief include:

Darvocet-N (acetaminophen and propoxyphene)—Schedule IV
Darvon Compound (aspirin and propoxyphene with caffeine to counteract the sedative effect of the narcotic)—Schedule IV
Empirin With Codeine No. 2 (aspirin and 15 mg codeine)—Schedule III
Empirin With Codeine No. 3 (aspirin and 30 mg codeine)—Schedule III
Empirin With Codeine No. 4 (aspirin and 60 mg codeine)—Schedule III
Percocet (acetaminophen and oxycodone)—Schedule II
Percodan (aspirin and oxycodone)—Schedule II
Tylenol With Codeine No. 1 (acetaminophen, 7.5 mg codeine)—Schedule III
Tylenol With Codeine No. 2 (acetaminophen, 15 mg codeine)—Schedule III
Tylenol With Codeine No. 3 (acetaminophen, 30 mg codeine)—Schedule III
Tylenol With Codeine No. 4 (acetaminophen, 60 mg codeine)—Schedule III

Vicodin (acetaminophen and hydrocodone)—Schedule III
Wygesic (acetaminophen and propoxyphene)—Schedule IV

Nonsteroidal Anti-Inflammatory Drugs (NSAID)

NSAIDs have analgesic effects and also inhibit the production of prostaglandins, but they have slightly less tendency to cause gastrointestinal side effects such as ulcers. They are similar enough to aspirin structurally that patients allergic to aspirin cannot be given NSAIDs. Nonsteroidal anti-inflammatory drugs include:

diclofenac (Voltaren)
fenoprofen (Nalfon)
flurbiprofen (Ansaid)
ibuprofen (Advil, Medipren, Nuprin)—over-the-counter
    (Motrin, Rufen)—prescription
ketoprofen (Orudis)
ketorolac (Toradol)
meclofenamate (Meclomen)
naproxen (Anaprox, Naprosyn)
piroxicam (Feldene)
sulindac (Clinoril)
tolmetin (Tolectin)

Note: Ketorolac (Toradol) is the only NSAID which is currently approved for I.M. administration.

The following NSAIDs are still investigational:

carprofen (Rimadyl)
etodolac (Ultradol)
isoxicam (Maxicam)

Note: The ending *-profen* is common to some generic nonsteroidal anti-inflammatory drugs.

One of the single largest uses for the nonsteroidal anti-inflammatory agents listed above is in treating the symptoms of arthritis. See Chapter 14, page 69.

Drugs for Migraine Headaches

The pain of migraine headaches is caused by constricted and then dilated blood vessels in the brain. Drugs which prevent or treat this pain act in several different ways.

Levels of serotonin, a vasoconstrictor, are increased before migraine attacks, and then decreased during the attack, causing vasodilation. The drug methysergide (Sansert) acts at serotonin receptor sites during a migraine attack to keep the blood vessels constricted.

Other drugs act on alpha receptors in the walls of cranial arteries to produce vasoconstriction:

ergotamine (Ergostat)
dihydroergotamine (D.H.E. 45)

Other drugs for migraine include beta blocking drugs. Their exact mechanism of action is not currently known. These drugs include:

atenolol (Tenormin)
metoprolol (Lopressor)
nadolol (Corgard)
propranolol (Inderal)
timolol (Blocadren)

Other drugs for the prevention of migraine headaches include calcium channel blockers:

nimodipine (Nimotop)
verapamil (Calan, Isoptin)

Combination drugs for migraine headaches. The following drugs contain ergotamine and also caffeine, which acts as a vasoconstrictor.

Cafergot
Wigraine

Miscellaneous Drugs

acetylcysteine (Mucomyst)   Used as an antidote for acetaminophen overdose, this drug acts to protect the liver, the main site of symptoms from acetaminophen toxicity.

Equagesic   A combination analgesic containing aspirin and the anti-anxiety drug meprobamate.

Fiorinal   A combination analgesic containing aspirin, caffeine, and a barbiturate for sedation.

flupirtine   An investigational non-narcotic analgesic.

methadone (Dolophine)   A narcotic drug used to treat addicts going through withdrawal from heroin. Methadone is addictive but it produces none of the euphoria of heroin. It prevents addicts from suffering severe heroin withdrawal symptoms, but they remain mentally alert and capable of benefitting from counseling and training. Methadone is given by mouth in an individualized dosage which is gradually tapered.

misoprostol (Cytotec)   Given to patients on long-term aspirin or nonsteroidal anti-inflammatory drugs to prevent the common side effect of stomach ulcer. Aspirin and NSAIDs inhibit the formation of prostaglandins that cause pain and inflammation. However, prostaglandins also normally act to protect the integrity of the stomach lining. Misoprostol is a synthetic prostaglandin which acts to protect the stomach when natural prostaglandin is inhibited in patients taking aspirin or NSAIDs.

naloxone (Narcan)   This drug is a narcotic antagonist and is used to reverse the effects of narcotic overdose, particularly that of respiratory depression. It competes for the same receptor sites as narcotic drugs.

DID YOU KNOW? Acetylcysteine (Mucomyst) is also used to thin the thick mucus secretions associated with cystic fibrosis.

27

Anti-Infective Drugs

Systemic anti-infective drugs are used to treat infections of all of the major body systems: the eyes, brain, ears, heart, lungs, and various abdominal organs. Anti-infective drugs include all classes of antibiotics (penicillins, cephalosporins, aminoglycosides, tetracyclines, and others) as well as the sulfonamides.

Sulfonamides

These anti-infective drugs are not classified as antibiotics but they do inhibit the growth of bacteria in the following way. Some bacteria must manufacture folic acid which is essential to their metabolism. Sulfonamides interfere with this process and cause these bacteria to die. Human cells as well as certain bacteria which can utilize folic acid from outside the cell are not affected by sulfonamide drugs. Sulfonamides are effective against many gram-negative and gram-positive bacteria. Sulfonamides, often called **sulfa drugs,** include:

> sulfacytine (Renoquid)
> sulfadiazine (Microsulfon)
> sulfamethizole (Thiosulfil)
> sulfamethoxazole (Gantanol)
> sulfasalazine (Azulfidine)
> sulfisoxazole (Gantrisin)
> triple sulfa (Terfonyl)

Sulfonamides are commonly used to treat urinary tract infections and otitis media. Sulfasalazine (Azulfidine) is indicated only for the treatment of ulcerative colitis.

HISTORICAL NOTE: In 1934 a German researcher was screening chemicals for possible medicinal use. A red dye used to color cloth was tested. It seemed to cure streptococcal infections in mice. The researcher's daughter was dying of streptococcal septicemia from pricking her finger. In desperation, he injected her with the dye and she recovered. The red dye was converted in the body into the anti-infective agent sulfanilamide. For the discovery of the first anti-infective drug, he won the Nobel prize.

Penicillins

The penicillins comprise a group of antibiotics which can kill bacteria. They include both natural and semisynthetic drugs which share a common molecular structure of a **beta-lactam ring.** All penicillins act by interfering with the structure of the cell wall that surrounds bacteria, causing disruption of the intracellular contents and cell death. Human cells have a cell membrane but no cell wall so are not adversely affected by penicillins.

The various drugs in the penicillin group differ among themselves in the following ways:

• Inactivated by gastric acid (only penicillin G).

• Inactivated by **penicillinase** (an enzyme produced by penicillin-resistant bacteria). This enzyme is also known as **beta-lactamase** because it inactivates the penicillins by breaking their chemical structure at the site of the beta-lactam ring. All of the penicillins are inactivated by penicillinase except methicillin, nafcillin, oxacillin, cloxacillin, and dicloxacillin.

• Little antibiotic activity against gram-negative bacteria. Extended spectrum penicillins such as carbenicillin, ticarcillin, mezlocillin, piperacillin, and azlocillin are active against gram-negative bacteria as well as gram-positive bacteria like other penicillins.

Antibiotics of the penicillin group include:

     amdinocillin (Coactin)
     amoxicillin (Amoxil, Larotid, Trimox, Utimox)
     ampicillin (Amcill, Omnipen, Polycillin, Principen, Totacillin)
     azlocillin (Azlin)
     bacampicillin (Spectrobid)
     carbenicillin (Geopen, Pyopen)
     cloxacillin (Cloxapen, Tegopen)
     cyclacillin (Cyclapen-W)
     dicloxacillin (Dynapen, Pathocil)
     methicillin (Staphcillin)
     mezlocillin (Mezlin)
     nafcillin (Unipen)

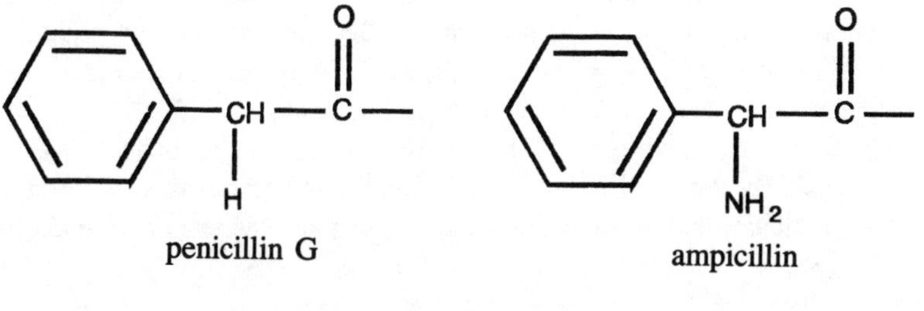

penicillin G   ampicillin

FIGURE 27-1
Detail of the chemical structure of penicillin G and ampicillin, showing the beta-lactam ring

oxacillin (Bactocill, Prostaphlin)
penicillin G
penicillin G benzathine (Bicillin, Permapen)
penicillin G potassium (Pentids)
penicillin G procaine (Duracillin, Wycillin)
penicillin V (V-Cillin K, Pen-Vee K)
piperacillin (Pipracil)
ticarcillin (Ticar)

HISTORICAL NOTE: In 1928 the Scottish bacteriologist, Alexander Fleming, concluded experiments looking for drugs which would inhibit the growth of staphylococcus. He left for a vacation and instructed an assistant to wash the culture plates which were soaking in the sink. When Fleming returned from vacation, the plates had not been washed. One culture plate had remained above the water and on it had grown a blue-green mold which clearly had killed the staphylococcus in a ring around it. Fleming identified this mold as *Penicillium notatum*; however, he was unable to extract a drug from it. (The mold itself contained only one part penicillin per two million parts mold.) He wrote a paper about his findings, but it remained unknown to the scientific world.

Work was halted on penicillin until the 1940s. In the meantime, the sulfonamide anti-infective drugs were discovered. During World War II, two researchers in England who were working with penicillin were afraid all of the supply would be destroyed in the bombing of London. Therefore, they smeared some of the mold inside their coat jackets and brought penicillin to the United States to be produced. A 43-year-old policeman was the first person to be injected with penicillin. He was dying of septicemia which had begun as an abscess when he scratched his face on a rosebush. Penicillin was in such short supply that his urine was saved each day and the penicillin in it extracted for the next day's dose. He was given the world's entire supply of penicillin. He responded well to the treatment, but on the fifth day the supply of penicillin ran out and he relapsed and died.

Penicillium notatum grew only on the surface of a culture media. It had to be produced in many shallow bottles and the yield was very small. Later, researchers found the strain *Penicillium chrysogenum* on a moldy cantaloupe in Peoria, Illinois. It was approximately 20 times more potent than the original culture and could be grown in larger quantities.

The first small amounts of commercially produced penicillin became available in 1942. By the end of that year, 100 patients had been treated with it. By 1945 penicillin had become a household word and the term *antibiotic* was coined as well.

Cephalosporins

The cephalosporins are made up of a group of antibiotics which can kill bacteria. They accomplish this by interfering with the structure of the cell wall which surrounds bacteria, causing disruption of intracellular contents and cell death. This group of antibiotics is further divided into first-, second-, and third-generation cephalosporins. This designation has nothing to do with when these antibiotics were discovered or first marketed, but instead divides them by their therapeutic antibiotic properties. First-generation cephalosporins are generally inactivated by bacteria which produce penicillinase, while third-generation cephalosporins show the greatest activity against resistant bacteria. In addition, the third-generation cephalosporins show greater activity against gram-negative bacteria in general.

First-generation cephalosporins include:

cefadroxil (Duricef, Ultracef)

cefazolin (Ancef, Kefzol)

cephalexin (Keflex, Keftab)

cephalothin (Keflin)

cephapirin (Cefadyl)

cephradine (Anspor, Velosef)

Second-generation cephalosporins include:

cefaclor (Ceclor)

cefamandole (Mandol)

cefmetazole (Zefazone)

cefonicid (Monocid)

ceforanide (Precef)

cefotetan (Cefotan)

cefoxitin (Mefoxin)

cefuroxime (Ceftin, Kefurox, Zinacef)

Third-generation cephalosporins include:

cefixime (Suprax)

cefoperazone (Cefobid)

cefotaxime (Claforan)

ceftazidime (Fortaz, Tazidime)

ceftizoxime (Cefizox)

ceftriaxone (Rocephin)

moxalactam (Moxam)

Note: Generic antibiotics beginning with *cefa* or *cepha* commonly belong to the cephalosporins. The spelling of these drugs must be checked carefully, as the generic names sound alike and can be confusing.

Cephalosporins and penicillins are structurally similar, and patients who are allergic to penicillin may have an allergic reaction if given cephalosporin antibiotics.

Aminoglycosides

The aminoglycosides comprise a group of antibiotics which kill bacteria. They do so by interfering with the synthesis of protein in the bacterial wall, causing disruption of intracellular contents and cell death. Aminoglycosides are primarily effective against gram-negative bacteria. Aminoglycosides given systemically include:

> amikacin (Amikin)
> gentamicin (Garamycin)
> kanamycin (Kantrex)
> netilmicin (Netromycin)
> tobramycin (Nebcin)

All aminoglycoside antibiotics have the potential to cause toxic effects to the auditory nerve (**ototoxicity**) and to the kidneys (**nephrotoxicity**). Patients on aminoglycosides are carefully monitored. However, because neomycin has the greatest incidence of toxicity, it is administered only as a topical antibiotic or given orally as an antibiotic bowel prep because it is not absorbed from the intestine. Kanamycin (Kantrex) is also used as a bowel prep in the same way.

Tetracyclines

The tetracyclines comprise a group of antibiotics which can inhibit bacteria. They do so by inhibiting the protein synthesis in the cell wall of bacteria. Tetracyclines are effective against both gram-positive and gram-negative bacteria. This group of drugs includes:

> demeclocycline (Declomycin)
> doxycycline (Vibramycin)
> methacycline (Rondomycin)
> minocycline (Minocin)
> oxytetracycline (Terramycin)
> tetracycline (Achromycin, Sumycin)

Note: The ending *-cycline* is common to generic tetracycline antibiotics.

The tetracyclines can cause permanent discoloration of the teeth; therefore, they are not prescribed for pregnant women (to protect the fetus' developing teeth) or for children.

Note: Antibiotics which are effective against both gram-negative and gram-positive bacteria are known as **broad-spectrum antibiotics.**

Combination Antibiotics

Augmentin   This drug contains amoxicillin combined with potassium clavulanate which can inactivate beta-lactamase enzymes produced by resistant bacteria.

Bactrim   A combination of trimethoprim (TMP), an antibiotic, and sulfamethoxazole (SMX, Gantanol), a sulfonamide anti-infective. This drug is used for urinary tract, respiratory tract, and ear infections. Another trade name for this combination is Septra. Bactrim DS is double-strength Bactrim.

Pediazole   A combination of erythromycin and the sulfa anti-infective sulfisoxazole (Gantrisin).

Primaxin This drug is a combination of the antibiotic imipenem, and cilastatin which inhibits the enzyme which metabolizes imipenem in the body. Primaxin is active against gram-negative and gram-positive bacteria.

Septra See *Bactrim*.

Timentin This drug is a combination of ticarcillin and potassium clavulanate. Clavulanate protects the ticarcillin from being metabolized by beta-lactamase enzymes like penicillinase before it has a chance to exert an antibiotic effect.

Unasyn This drug combines ampicillin with the drug sulbactam which can inactivate beta-lactamase enzymes like penicillinase produced by bacteria resistant to ampicillin.

Miscellaneous Antibiotic Drugs

aztreonam (Azactam) The first of the new class of **monobactam antibiotics**. This drug is effective against gram-negative bacteria.

chloramphenicol (Chloromycetin) This antibiotic is effective against both gram-negative and gram-positive bacteria and can cross the blood-brain barrier, but is reserved for treating serious infections because it can cause bone marrow depression.

ciprofloxacin (Cipro) This antibiotic is effective against gram-negative and gram-positive bacteria.

clindamycin (Cleocin) Effective against gram-positive bacteria, this drug is an alternative to penicillin for serious infections.

colistin (Coly-Mycin S) Effective against gram-negative bacteria, this drug is used to treat diarrhea and GI infections.

enoxacin (Comprecin) An investigational antibiotic related to ciprofloxacin.

erythromycin (E.E.S., E-Mycin, ERYC, Erypar, EryPed, Ery-Tab, Ilosone, Ilotycin, Pediamycin) This agent is the drug of choice for Mycoplasma pneumonia, Legionnaire disease, and infections caused by *Haemophilus influenzae*. It may also be used as an alternative to the penicillins or tetracyclines.

lincomycin (Lincocin) Effective against gram-positive and gram-negative bacteria, this drug is an alternative to penicillin for serious infections.

metronidazole (Flagyl) Effective against anaerobic bacteria.

novobiocin (Albamycin) Used for gram-positive infections when other antibiotics cannot be used.

probenecid A drug which helps to prolong the therapeutic blood levels of ampicillin by inhibiting its excretion into the urine.

troleandomycin (Tao) This drug is effective only against streptococcal infections.

vancomycin (Vancocin) This drug is used as an alternative to the penicillin and cephalosporin antibiotics, and is effective for resistant staphylococci.

28

AIDS Drugs/Antiviral Drugs

Drugs Used to Treat AIDS

Acquired immunodeficiency syndrome (AIDS) is a fatal disease in which the human immunodeficiency virus (HIV) enters helper T lymphocytes (a specific type of white blood cell of the immune system) and directs the lymphocyte to produce more HIV using its own DNA mechanism. Once this is accomplished, the white blood cell is destroyed. The newly produced viruses are released into the bloodstream to infect more helper T lymphocytes and further weaken the immune system. Although the body does produce antibodies against the virus, the immune system is never able to control or eradicate the disease.

With the breakdown of the immune system, the body is also unable to defend itself against other illnesses. Malignancies and secondary infections of *Pneumocystis carinii* pneumonia, herpes simplex virus, and *Candida albicans,* to name a few, quickly become life threatening.

Drug therapy for AIDS currently focuses on the use of antiviral agents to suppress the AIDS virus and other opportunistic viruses as well as drugs to treat the secondary illnesses mentioned above.

Antiviral Agents Used to Treat AIDS

At the present time, azidothymidine (AZT), now known as zidovudine (Retrovir), is the only drug approved by the FDA for treating AIDS. There are, however, many investigational antiviral drugs being tested for their effectiveness against HIV; some drugs already approved for treating other viruses are also being tested for their effectiveness against the AIDS virus. These drugs include:

acemannan (Carrisyn)
ampligen
ansamycin (Rifabutin)
dextran sulfate (Uendex)
dideoxycytidine (ddC)
dideoxyinosine (ddI)
foscarnet
interferon alfa-2a (Roferon-A)
interferon alfa-2b (Intron A)
interferon beta (Betaseron)

146

isoprinosine
Novapren
ribavirin (Virazole)
suramin

HISTORICAL NOTE: Azidothymidine (AZT) was originally synthesized in 1974. It was tested as a treatment for cancer but was not effective. Other uses for it were not investigated and it was simply "shelved."

In 1984, although there were only 3,000 reported cases of AIDS in the United States, researchers at the National Cancer Institute, including the co-discoverer of the AIDS virus, Dr. Robert Gallo, approached Burroughs Wellcome pharmaceutical company to develop a drug to treat AIDS. Although other pharmaceutical companies were also approached, their concern about working with the deadly virus as well as the apparently limited use for the drug at that time resulted in an unenthusiastic response. Burroughs Wellcome, however, accepted and tested many different drugs, one of which was azidothymidine (AZT).

In 1986 clinical testing of azidothymidine was begun, using a double-blind study in which severely ill AIDS patients were divided into two groups: one group received AZT while the control group received a placebo. Shortly after the study was begun, it was ended when it was found that those in the control group had a 40% mortality rate while those receiving AZT had only a 6% mortality rate. In March 1988, just four months after a new drug application was filed, the FDA gave its final approval to AZT, the shortest period of time such approval ever required.

As the exclusive manufacturer and distributor, Burroughs Wellcome chose the generic name zidovudine for this new AIDS drug, and the trade name Retrovir. The trade name refers to the fact that the AIDS virus belongs to a class of viruses known as retroviruses.

Miscellaneous Drugs Used to Treat AIDS

lithium (Eskalith, Lithobid, Lithotabs) The drug of choice for treating manic-depressive disorders, lithium has the known side effect of causing leukocytosis (increased white blood cell count). This becomes a desirable therapeutic effect in AIDS patients whose white blood cells are destroyed by HIV.

AIDS vaccine In early 1988, the National Institutes of Health began to develop an AIDS vaccine. This still experimental vaccine consists of purified protein derived from genetic material from the AIDS virus which is reproduced using recombinant DNA technology. This material stimulates the body to produce antibodies against the AIDS virus but, because it contains only pieces of HIV, the vaccine itself cannot cause AIDS.

pentamidine (NebuPent) In an aerosolized form, this drug is inhaled and concentrates in the alveoli. It is used to treat *Pneumocystis carinii* pneumonia. Its advantage is that it does not produce as many side effects as pentamidine taken orally.

pentamidine (Pentam 300) This oral antiprotozoal drug is used to treat *Pneumocystis carinii*, an opportunistic pathogen which frequently causes pneumonia in AIDS patients.

nystatin (Mycostatin) An antifungal/antiyeast agent, this drug is used to treat yeast infections caused by *Candida albicans* in the mouth of immunocompromised AIDS patients. This oral infection is alternatively known as oral candidiasis, monilia, or thrush. The drug is applied topically as a solution (the patient is told to "swish and swallow") or as a troche (lozenge).

Other Antiviral Drugs

Other antiviral drugs are used to treat severe viral infections such as those caused by the following:

      respiratory syncytial virus (RSV), treated with ribavirin (Virazole)

      influenza virus A, treated with

         amantadine (Symmetrel)

         ribavirin (Virazole)

         rimantadine (Flumadine)—an investigational drug

      herpes simplex virus, treated with

         acyclovir (Zovirax)

         ribavirin (Virazole)

         vidarabine (Ara-A, Vira-A)

      cytomegalovirus (CMV), treated with

         ganciclovir (Cytovene)

Topical Antiviral Drugs

Topical drugs used to treat viral infections of the skin are discussed in Chapter 11, page 54.

REVIEW QUESTIONS

1. Define these abbreviations: AIDS, HIV, AZT, RSV, CMV.
2. What two distinct and very different medical uses does the drug lithium have?

SPELLING TIPS

- interferon alfa-2a and interferon alfa-2b (An unusual spelling of the Greek term alpha.)

29

Antifungal Drugs

Fungi are generally opportunistic organisms which can cause disease topically or systemically. In immunocompromised patients, their effects can be quite serious. Topical fungal infections include ringworm, athlete's foot, and jock itch, and the topical drugs used to treat these infections are discussed in Chapter 11. However, a fungal infection of the nails (onychomycosis) can be difficult to treat topically. For that condition, as well as for far more serious systemic fungal infections such as cryptococcal meningitis, lung infections, and coccidioidomycosis, oral or intravenous antifungal drugs are necessary. These drugs include:

amphotericin B (Fungizone)
fluconazole (Diflucan)
flucytosine (Ancobon)
griseofulvin (Fulvicin, Grifulvin, Grisactin)
ketoconazole (Nizoral)
miconazole (Monistat i.v.)

DID YOU KNOW? The new antifungal drug fluconazole (Diflucan) costs more than nine dollars per tablet.

Yeasts, such as *Candida albicans,* are often classified as fungi. The drugs used to treat topical yeast infections of the mouth (thrush) are discussed in Chapter 19. Drugs used to treat vaginal yeast infections are discussed in Chapter 23. Systemic yeast infections due to *Candida* can be treated orally or intravenously with all of the antifungal drugs mentioned above with the exception of griseofulvin which is not active against *Candida.*

30

Chemotherapy Drugs

A neoplasm is a new growth of cells which may be either malignant or benign. All malignant neoplasms are referred to as cancers, from a Latin word meaning *crab,* because cancers metastasize or spread outward from the original site like the legs of a crab. Uncontrolled cell division and metastasis are identifying characteristics of cancerous cells.

"Cancer cells are the anarchists of the body, for they know no law, pay no regard for the commonwealth, serve no useful function, and cause disharmony and death in their surrounds," wrote William Boyd, in *An Introduction to the Study of Disease,* 1971, as quoted by Michael C. Gerald, *Pharmacology: An Introduction to Drugs,* 2d ed. (Englewood Cliffs, N.J.: Prentice-Hall, Inc., 1981), p. 574.

As cancerous cells invade normal tissues and organs, function is impaired to the point of causing death unless treatment with surgery, radiation, or chemotherapy drugs can intervene.

In order to properly treat any type of cancer, the physician must determine two things: the type of cancer and the stage. To determine the type of cancer, a biopsy is taken from the tumor site or a blood specimen is drawn for examination of cells. Only when the exact type of cancer can be specified by the pathologist will the physician select an appropriate chemotherapy regimen.

In addition to the type of cancer, the physician must also know the extent of the cancer before beginning treatment. The extent of cancer progression is referred to as the stage. In general, stage I cancer has not spread beyond the primary site, while stage II cancer has metastasized to regional lymph nodes. The selection of various chemotherapy drugs and protocols is based on the pathologic diagnosis and also the stage of that cancer. A treatment which would be appropriate for one type of cancer in stage I might not be appropriate for the same type of cancer at a more advanced stage. Indeed, all types of prostatic cancer do not respond equally well to chemotherapy; some types are treated by radiation alone.

Chemotherapy drugs are most effective when initiated at the early stages of cancer when there are fewer cancer cells present in the body. "At the time of diagnosis of acute leukemia, one trillion cancer cells are generally present and widely distributed throughout the body of the [patient]. If an antileukemic agent were able to kill 99.9 percent of the cells present, patients would show symptomatic improvement although they would still harbor one billion cancer cells." (Gerald, p. 581.)

150

The term *adjuvant therapy* is taken from a Latin word meaning *aiding*. Adjuvant therapy refers to chemotherapy (or radiation therapy) which is given to cancer patients after they have had surgery to remove a tumor. The purpose of adjuvant therapy is to deal with any tumor cells remaining.

A remission occurs when cancerous cells stop actively reproducing. Some cancer patients experience a complete remission following chemotherapy, others have a partial **remission,** and some actually have tumor growth while being treated with chemotherapy. When tumor size increases or new metastatic lesions appear despite chemotherapy, the patient is said to have failed chemotherapy. A new combination of chemotherapeutic drugs may then be tried. If no drugs are suitable for therapy, the patient may be offered palliative chemotherapy or radiation therapy to provide temporary relief only.

HISTORICAL NOTE: In the early 1900s, the only treatments available for tumorous cancers were surgical excision and radiation therapy. The discovery of the first chemotherapy drug came about serendipitously. During the 1940s, researchers reviewing records from World War I noticed that Allied soldiers who were exposed to the chemical weapon nitrogen mustard gas had a decreased level of white blood cells. It was thought that this might be used to therapeutic effect in patients with leukemia whose white cell counts are elevated. Nitrogen mustard and its derivatives are still used to treat leukemia today.

Categories of Chemotherapy Drugs
1. **Antimetabolites.** As a group, antimetabolites compete with endogenous substances necessary for cell metabolism and DNA synthesis. Acting as antagonists, antimetabolites take the place of necessary chemicals within a cell while also blocking the necessary substance from entering the cell. As the cell is unable to properly continue metabolism, it eventually dies. There are several subcategories of antimetabolite chemotherapy drugs. These include:
* **Purine antagonists.** Purine is a general term referring to several component chemicals of DNA. Purine antagonists block the use of one of the purine components by DNA to prevent cell division. Chemotherapy drugs which block purine include:
> mercaptopurine (Purinethol)
> thioguanine
* **Pyrimidine antagonists.** Pyrimidine is a general term referring to several component chemicals of DNA. Pyrimidine antagonists block the use of the pyrimidine components by DNA to prevent cell division. Chemotherapy drugs which block pyrimidine include:
> cytarabine (Ara-C, Cytosar-U)
> fluorouracil (5-fluorouracil, 5-FU, Adrucil)
> floxuridine (FUDR)

DID YOU KNOW? The development of cytarabine was based on a substance found in Caribbean sea sponges.

• **Folic acid antagonists.** The B vitamin folic acid is required for the synthesis of both purines and pyrimidines which are later used to form DNA and RNA. Chemotherapy drugs which block the uptake of folic acid by cells include **methotrexate (Folex).**

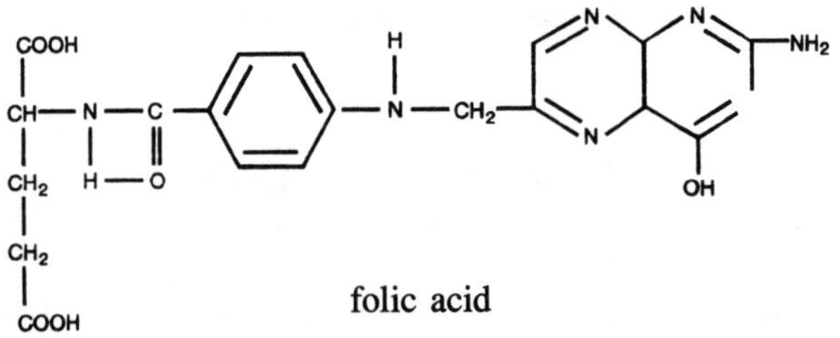

folic acid

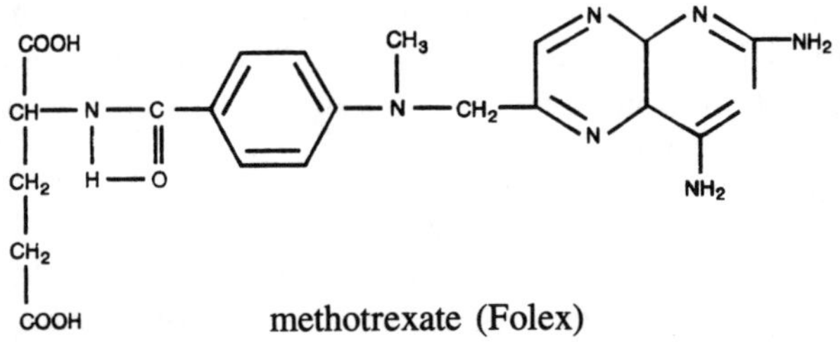

methotrexate (Folex)

FIGURE 30-1
Chemical structure of folic acid and the folic acid antagonist drug, methotrexate (Folex)

2. **Alkylating agents.** Alkylation refers to a chemical substitution which occurs when an alkyl group from the chemotherapy drug's molecular structure is substituted for a hydrogen molecule on the DNA strand. This causes the DNA strands to break apart or to bind together incorrectly. The cell is then unable to divide properly. All alkylating agents are derivatives of nitrogen mustard. Chemotherapy drugs which act as alkylating agents include:

> busulfan (Myleran)
> carboplatin (Paraplatin)
> carmustine (BiCNU)
> chlorambucil (Leukeran)
> cisplatin (cis-platinum, Platinol)

cyclophosphamide (Cytoxan)
ifosfamide (Ifex)
lomustine (CeeNu)
mechlorethamine (nitrogen mustard, Mustargen)
melphalan (Alkeran)
pipobroman (Vercyte)
streptozocin (Zanosar)
thiotepa
uracil mustard

3. Chemotherapeutic antibiotics. Most antibiotics act only on the cell wall of bacteria. Human cells, which do not have a cell wall (only a cell membrane), are not affected by standard antibiotics. However, a special class of antibiotics are used as chemotherapy drugs. They do affect human cells. All of the chemotherapeutic antibiotics act on DNA to inhibit synthesis of it or to break or bind DNA strands so that cell division cannot be completed. Chemotherapeutic antibiotics are never used to treat bacterial infections. Chemotherapeutic antibiotics include:

bleomycin (Blenoxane)
dactinomycin (actinomycin D, Cosmegen)
daunorubicin (Cerubidine)
doxorubicin (Adriamycin, Rubrex)
mitomycin (Mutamycin)
mitoxantrone (Novantrone)
plicamycin (Mithracin)

4. Hormonal agents. Certain tumors, specifically those arising from tissue influenced by the hormones estrogen and progesterone/androgen show regression when treated with a drug which produces the opposite hormonal effect/environment. For example, estrogen given to a patient with testicular cancer changes the favorable hormonal environment provided by endogenous androgens (male hormones) and causes the tumor cells to die. Hormonal drugs used to treat breast cancer include androgens/progestins and estrogen blocking drugs such as:

medroxyprogesterone (Depo-Provera)
megestrol (Megace)
tamoxifen (Nolvadex)
testolactone (Teslac)

Hormonal drugs used to treat prostatic cancer include estrogen or androgen-blocking drugs such as:

diethylstilbestrol (Stilphostrol)
estramustine (Emcyt)
flutamide (Eulexin)
goserelin (Zoladex)
leuprolide (Lupron)
polyestradiol (Estradurin)

5. **Mitotic inhibiting agents.** Mitotic inhibiting drugs act during a very specific point in cell division known as metaphase which occurs just before the chromosomes divide and migrate to each end of the cell. Mitotic inhibiting drugs stop metaphase and prevent any of the subsequent steps of cell division. Mitotic inhibiting drugs used for chemotherapy include:

> etoposide (VP-16, VePesid)
> vinblastine (Velban)
> vincristine (Oncovin)
> vindesine (Eldisine)—an investigational drug

DID YOU KNOW? Vincristine, vinblastine, and vindesine are derived from the periwinkle plant. Another common name for this evergreen ground cover is vinca. It takes over six tons of periwinkle leaves to produce one ounce of these drugs. Etoposide is a semisynthetic derivative of the May apple plant.

Chemotherapy Protocols

Chemotherapy protocols were introduced in the late 1960s in order to combine the effectiveness of several drugs against one specific type of cancer. Prior to this, only single agent chemotherapy drugs were used. In combining the drugs of a chemotherapy protocol, the success of each drug in treating a certain type of cancer is compared to that of others. The most successful drugs are combined into one protocol to maximize the effectiveness of therapy through various mechanisms of action but also to minimize the side effects caused by large doses of just one drug. Today, chemotherapy protocols are used to treat nearly every type of cancer.

Protocols are designated by acronyms which combine the first letter of either the generic name, trade name, or abbreviation of each drug in the protocol. For example:

Protocol Name	*Drug*
MOPP	Mustargen (nitrogen mustard)
	Oncovin (vincristine)
	procarbazine (Matulane)
	prednisone

Corticosteroids

Corticosteroids such as prednisone and dexamethasone are often given with chemotherapy drugs to decrease inflammation in healthy tissues. See Chapter 21.

Antiemetics

Because of their effect on rapidly dividing cells, chemotherapy drugs may damage the lining cells of the GI tract and may also cause nausea and vomiting. Antiemetic drugs used to treat this are described in Chapter 13, page 67.

Miscellaneous Chemotherapy Agents

asparaginase (Elspar)   Used only with other chemotherapy agents to treat lympho-cytic leukemia. This drug is an enzyme derived from the common intestinal bacteria *Escherichia coli (E. coli)*. It acts by destroying the amino acid asparagine. Asparagine is not one of the eight essential amino acids needed by the body to produce protein. Normal human cells can synthesize their own supply of aspara-gine. Leukemic cells, however, cannot synthesize asparagine. By destroying asparagine and cutting off the supply this drug selectively kills leukemic cells.

dacarbazine (DTIC-Dome)   Used only to treat malignant melanoma.

hydroxyurea (Hydrea)   This drug inhibits an enzyme which must react with purines or pyrimidines in order for normal cell division to occur.

interferon   Interferon is a natural body substance which is released when a cell is invaded by a virus. It then stimulates surrounding cells to produce certain pro-teins which prevent the virus from spreading. In the 1960s, in an "episode of the popular adventure series Flash Gordon, a spaceman infected with an extrater-restrial virus was saved by injections of interferon." ("Interferon: Trying to Live Up to Its Press," *FDA Consumer,* Nov. 1981. Rockville, Md.: Department of Health and Human Services, p. 1.)

At one point, it was hoped that interferon would be the magic cure for the common cold caused by viruses, but its cost was prohibitively expensive. All interferons today are manufactured by recombinant DNA technology and are used to treat viral diseases and many neoplastic diseases.

> interferon alfa-2a (Roferon-A)
> interferon alfa-2b (Intron A)
> interferon alfa-n3 (Alferon N)

L-asparaginase   See *asparaginase.*

levamisole (Ergamisol)   Used only in combination with fluorouracil for colon cancer.

procarbazine (Matulane)   Used only in combination with other chemotherapy agents to treat Hodgkin disease.

REVIEW QUESTIONS

1. What are the five main categories of chemotherapy drugs?
2. Why do some chemotherapy drugs so commonly cause the side effect of severe nausea and vomiting? (Also, see page 67 for more information.)

31

Anesthetics

Anesthesia may be defined as the absence of feeling, sensation, or pain. Anesthesia may be obtained on the skin (by topical application of anesthetic drugs), in the skin and deeper tissues (by subcutaneous local injection), in one body part (by regional nerve block), or in the trunk and lower extremities (by epidural, caudal, or spinal anesthesia). Topical, local, regional, and epidural/spinal anesthesia are all obtained by blocking the flow of sodium ions across the nerve cell membrane, thereby blocking the production and conduction of a nerve impulse which conveys the message of pain.

General anesthesia involves a loss of consciousness which produces total body anesthesia during surgical procedures.

Historical Notes on Anesthesia

The first mention of general anesthesia was in Genesis, the first book of the Bible, when God caused a deep sleep to fall on Adam prior to creating Eve. But for centuries, the only pain relief available to much of the world was from the use of alcohol or opium. These drugs failed to produce complete anesthesia, and many surgeries were performed quickly with assistants holding the patient.

In 1772 **nitrous oxide** (N_2O) was discovered. Rather than being administered as an anesthetic, it was used at social parties to produce euphoria and was commonly known as laughing gas. Nitrous oxide was not recognized as a general anesthetic until the 1860s.

During the first half of the 1800s, then, surgery was still performed without the benefit of general anesthesia. During the PBS television series "Treasure Houses of Great Britain," the story was told of the Marquis de Angelcy, whose leg was destroyed by cannon shot during the battle of Waterloo (1815). His leg was sawed off. The surgeon wrote afterwards that he was amazed that the patient's pulse did not vary during the operation. The Marquis' only recorded comment was, "I do not think the saw was very sharp."

In 1846 William Morton, a Boston dentist, recognized that **ether** could produce a general anesthesia. He gave the first public demonstration of surgery performed under ether anesthesia at Massachusetts General Hospital. The term *anesthesia* was coined at that time to describe the effects of ether. A monument at Morton's grave reads:

> Inventor and Revealer of Anaesthetic Inhalation.
> Before Whom, in All Time, Surgery was Agony.
> By Whom, Pain in Surgery Was Averted and Annulled.
> Since Whom, Science Has Control of Pain.
>
> Alfred G. Gilman and Louis S. Goodman, et al.,
> *The Pharmacologic Basis of Therapeutics,* 7th ed.
> (New York: Macmillan Publishing Co., 1985), p. 261

From its first use in 1846, ether enjoyed great popularity as a general anesthetic. However, its use presented several drawbacks. It had an extremely unpleasant odor when inhaled, it was highly explosive, and it frequently produced severe postoperative vomiting. Its use was discontinued in the 1960s.

At approximately the same time that ether was discovered, the Scottish obstetrician James Simpson introduced the general anesthetic **chloroform.** Chloroform had two advantages over ether: a more pleasant odor and it was not explosive. However, it was much more toxic and its use was associated with a higher mortality rate. It was used little after World War I.

Thus within the scope of 17 years, the first three general anesthetics—ether, chloroform, and **nitrous oxide**—were introduced. Today, only nitrous oxide is still in use.

For centuries, the South American Indians chewed the leaves of the coca bush for their euphoric effect. Cocaine was derived from these leaves. It was recognized as a topical anesthetic in 1880 and still has limited use as such. For many years, synthetic substitutes for cocaine were sought. This resulted in the production of **procaine (Novocain)**, the prototype of local anesthetics.

In 1920 the technique of endotracheal intubation was perfected which allowed greater control of patient ventilation and anesthetic administration.

In 1929 the fourth general anesthetic, **cyclopropane**, was discovered by accident during research on another chemical. It was used widely until the late 1950s, when its use was curtailed due to the danger of explosion in operating rooms that contained more and more electrical equipment.

In 1935 **thiopental (Pentothal)**, a barbiturate, was given I.V. and was found to rapidly induce general anesthesia. It is still used today.

For centuries, the South American Indians had used arrows dipped in curare for hunting animals and in battle. This drug causes death by muscle paralysis. It was unknown to the rest of the world until 1595, when Sir Walter Raleigh brought it to England. Not until the 1940s, however, was **curare** introduced as the first neuromuscular blocking agent used with general anesthesia. Up until that time, abdominal surgery presented a challenge to both the surgeon and the anesthesiologist because the abdominal muscles remained taut and unyielding except under the deepest general anesthesia. With curare, the anesthesiologist could maintain a lighter level of anesthesia while still obtaining complete abdominal wall relaxation. Other neuromuscular blocking agents were later developed.

In 1948 **lidocaine (Xylocaine),** the most widely used topical, local, regional, and spinal anesthetic, was introduced.

No further advances were made in anesthetics until 1956, when **halothane (Fluothane)** was developed from technology arising from research with fluorine which had been conducted with uranium during World War II to produce the atomic bomb. This drug marked the beginning of a new category of inhaled general anesthetic agents which are still used today.

Topical Anesthetic Agents

Topical anesthetics provide brief periods of anesthesia to a limited depth on the skin. Local anesthetics are used to provide temporary symptomatic relief for various skin disorders including minor burns, sunburn, rashes, insect bites, etc. These drugs include:

benzocaine (Americaine, Dermoplast, Solarcaine)
dibucaine (Nupercainal)
lidocaine (Xylocaine)
pramoxine (Tronothane)
tetracaine (Pontocaine)

Topical anesthetics used on the mucous membranes of the mouth and throat are discussed in Chapter 19.

Local Anesthetic Agents

Local anesthetics provide brief periods of anesthesia in small, localized areas of the skin and adjacent tissues following administration by subcutaneous injection. Local anesthetics are used in dental procedures and for minor surgical procedures and biopsies.

Drugs used as local anesthetics include:
bupivacaine (Marcaine)
chloroprocaine (Nesacaine)
lidocaine (Xylocaine)
mepivacaine (Carbocaine)
procaine (Novocain)

The local anesthetic lidocaine (Xylocaine) is available with or without **epinephrine (Adrenalin)** in the solution. Epinephrine (Adrenalin) is a powerful vasoconstrictor which decreases blood flow to the tissue where it is injected. This therapeutic action controls bleeding and also prolongs the anesthetic action of lidocaine. The use of locally injected epinephrine (Adrenalin) is contraindicated in certain areas of the body, such as the tip of the nose, fingers, toes, or ears, because the blood supply is limited and excessive local vasoconstriction would lead to necrosis and skin sloughing. In these areas, lidocaine (Xylocaine) without epinephrine is used for local anesthesia.

Nerve Block Anesthetic Agents

Several anesthetic agents are given via subcutaneous injection directly near a particular nerve plexus (group of nerves) and its branches. This directly blocks all impulses and is known as **regional anesthesia** or nerve block anesthesia. For example, the brachial plexus can be injected to provide anesthesia of the upper extremity for surgery in that region.

Drugs used to produce nerve block regional anesthesia include:
bupivacaine (Marcaine)
chloroprocaine (Nesacaine)
etidocaine (Duranest)
lidocaine (Xylocaine)
mepivacaine (Carbocaine)
procaine (Novocain)

Spinal and Epidural Anesthetic Agents

Spinal anesthesia involves the injection of an anesthetic agent into the subarachnoid space between the vertebrae of the lumbar region. Epidural anesthesia involves the injection of an anesthetic agent into the epidural space; the drug then moves into the subarachnoid space to produce anesthesia.

Drugs used to produce spinal or epidural anesthesia include:
bupivacaine (Marcaine)
etidocaine (Duranest)
lidocaine (Xylocaine)
procaine (Novocain)
tetracaine (Pontocaine)

Note: The ending -*caine* is common to generic anesthetic agents with the exception of those used to produce general anesthesia.

General Anesthetic Agents

General anesthesia involves the loss of consciousness to produce anesthesia, a technique which distinguishes it from all other types of anesthesia. In the operating room, the patient is first given a drug to induce general anesthesia. Once the patient is unconscious and intubated, then other anesthetic agents are given to maintain general anesthesia. Drugs for **induction of anesthesia** are generally given intravenously; drugs used to maintain general anesthesia may be given intravenously or by inhalation.

Intravenous agents for the induction of general anesthesia. These intravenous drugs provide a rapid loss of consciousness to avoid patient anxiety and quickly initiate anesthesia. Drugs which induce general anesthesia include ultrashort-acting barbiturates and other nonbarbiturate agents. All of the ultrashort-acting barbiturates are classified as Schedule III or IV drugs, but the short duration of their use as induction anesthetics limits their addictive potential.

Ultrashort-acting barbiturates:
    methohexital (Brevital)
    thiamylal (Surital)
    thiopental (Pentothal)
Nonbarbiturate agents:
    etomidate (Amidate)
    ketamine (Ketalar)
    midazolam (Versed)
Note: Midazolam (Versed) may also be given preoperatively to produce sedation and amnesia.

Inhaled anesthetic agents for maintenance of general anesthesia. Anesthetic drugs in the form of a gas may be inhaled to maintain general anesthesia. These drugs include:
    enflurane (Ethrane)
    halothane (Fluothane)
    isoflurane (Forane)
    methoxyflurane (Penthrane)
    nitrous oxide (N_2O)

Intravenous anesthetic agents for maintenance of general anesthesia. Drugs used alone or in combination with inhaled anesthetics to maintain general anesthesia include narcotic analgesics which bind with opiate receptors in the brain to block pain and maintain unconsciousness. All of these drugs are narcotics with a Schedule II classification, but the short duration of their use as general anesthetics limits their addictive potential.
    alfentanil (Alfenta)
    fentanyl (Sublimaze)
    sufentanil (Sufenta)

Neuromuscular Blocking Agents
Used During General Anesthesia

Neuromuscular blocking agents are given intravenously to block nerve transmissions throughout the body to induce skeletal muscle relaxation. This is particularly important during abdominal surgery when the abdominal muscles must relax to provide adequate visualization of the operative field. Neuromuscular blocking agents include:
    atracurium (Tracrium)
    gallamine triethiodide (Flaxedil)
    metocurine (Metubine)
    pancuronium (Pavulon)
    succinylcholine (Anectine, Sucostrin)
    tubocurarine
    vecuronium (Norcuron)

Miscellaneous Drugs Used During Surgery

atropine Given I.M. preoperatively, this anticholinergic drug blocks the action of acetylcholine. This produces the desirable effects of decreased mouth and upper airway secretions as well as relaxation of the smooth muscle of the larynx—both of which facilitate endotracheal intubation.

diazepam (Valium) A preoperative medication given I.M. or I.V. to decrease anxiety and provide sedation. A sufficient dosage will also produce amnesia. This is useful during minor surgical/dental procedures and endoscopies, as general anesthesia can be avoided and yet the patient is still able to respond to commands to facilitate the procedure.

dantrolene (Dantrium) This drug is used to treat malignant hyperthermia, a rare but life-threatening systemic reaction that occurs in some patients undergoing general anesthesia. It is due to a genetic defect which causes the release of massive amounts of calcium from muscle cells. Dantrolene keeps the muscle from releasing calcium.

droperidol (Inapsine) A sedative given I.V. preoperatively or during surgery to decrease anxiety.

hydroxyzine (Vistaril) A preoperative medication given I.M. to produce sedation, relieve anxiety, and decrease nausea and vomiting.

Innovar A combination of fentanyl and droperidol which reduces anxiety and decreases motor activity during surgical procedures in which the patient is conscious.

meperidine (Demerol) A narcotic drug given I.M. preoperatively to decrease the sensation of pain and provide sedation.

mephentermine (Wyamine) A vasopressor drug used specifically to treat the hypotension that can occur during spinal anesthesia.

metaraminol (Aramine) A vasopressor drug used specifically to treat the hypotension that can occur during spinal anesthesia.

methoxamine (Vasoxyl) A vasopressor drug used specifically to treat the hypotension that can occur during spinal anesthesia.

32

Intravenous Fluids and Blood Products

Intravenous fluid therapy may be instituted for one of several reasons:
- To correct body fluid imbalance
- To correct decreased levels of electrolytes or glucose
- To administer drugs
- To administer blood or blood products
- To provide nutritional support
- To maintain venous access between drug doses

Intravenous therapy may be ordered in various ways. An intravenous (I.V.) line includes a bag or bottle containing I.V. fluid, connecting tubing, and a needle or flexible catheter inserted in the vein. Additional equipment may include a machine which automatically infuses a set amount of fluid (ml/hr. or drops/minute). The injection of a single dose of a drug (bolus) may be given through a port (rubber stopper) in the connecting tubing. This method is referred to as **I.V. push,** as the drug is pushed in slowly by hand. A drug may also be mixed with the fluid in an I.V. bag or bottle and administered continuously over several hours. This is known as **I.V. drip.** Finally, a drug may be mixed in a very small I.V. bag or bottle connected into the I.V. tubing, to run in over an hour or less. This method is known as **I.V. piggyback.**

A **heparin lock** is a special type of device for intravenous access. It contains a small reservoir which holds heparin and keeps the vein free of clots without the use of I.V. fluids. It is used to administer drugs on an intermittent basis. Following drug administration, the reservoir is again filled with heparin.

Intravenous Fluids

The most commonly used intravenous fluids contain dextrose or electrolytes or a combination of both.

Glucose, a simple sugar, is the only carbohydrate the cells can use for an energy source. Although the food we eat contains complex sugars such as sucrose (table sugar) and complex carbohydrates (starches), the body must first metabolize them to glucose before they can be utilized.

I.V. fluids contain dextrose rather than glucose. Dextrose is the dextrorotary isomer of glucose and acts in the bloodstream in the same way as glucose.

A dextrose and water combination forms the basis for many intravenous solutions. Frequently used concentrations include:

dextrose 5% in water (D-5-W)

dextrose 10% in water (D-10-W)

dextrose 50% in water (D-50-W)

Dextrose 50% in water is used only in emergencies when blood sugar levels fall so low as to be life-threatening. This severe hypoglycemia can occur in diabetics and premature infants.

If dextrose is not needed, often an intravenous solution of sodium and water will be administered. Sodium is an important electrolyte in both intracellular and extracellular fluids in the body. The intravenous solution contains sodium and water in proportions which parallel those in tissue fluids. This concentration is known as a physiologic salt solution or normal saline. Normal saline (NS) actually equals a 0.9% solution of sodium chloride and water. Sometimes an I.V. solution of half normal saline is ordered; this is written as 0.45% rather than 0.5%.

normal saline (NS)   0.9% NaCl

half normal saline   0.45% NaCl

Frequently dextrose and normal saline are combined into a single solution such as:

dextrose 5% in normal saline (D5/NS)

Lactated Ringer's solution is a combination intravenous fluid containing fixed amounts of dextrose, sodium, potassium, calcium, chloride, and lactate. It was named for the English physiologist, Sidney Ringer.

lactated Ringer's (LR)

Ringer's lactate (RL)

dextrose 5% in lactated Ringer's (D5/LR)

Crystalloid is a general term used to describe intravenous solutions which provide normal saline with or without other electrolytes.

Dextrose and electrolyte intravenous fluids are used to maintain fluid and electrolyte balance and supply calories, but they are unable to completely meet long-term nutritional needs. Specifically, they lack protein, fat, and vitamins. Patients whose nutritional needs cannot be met with dextrose and electrolyte fluids may be given a specially prepared intravenous solution known as **total parenteral nutrition (TPN).** This is prepared in the hospital pharmacy and is individually tailored for each patient according to the physician's orders. It contains specific amounts of essential amino acids (protein), as well as electrolytes, vitamins, and minerals. To meet fat requirements, a separate intravenous solution of lipids may also be given. These lipid solutions contain fat in the form of soybean or safflower oil along with water, glycerin, and egg yolk. Lipids are a more concentrated source of calories than dextrose and also contain essential fatty acids.

intravenous lipids (Intralipid, Liposyn, NutriLipid)

A specially formulated combination of twelve vitamins for intravenous administration is **multiple vitamin complex for injection** (M.V.C. 9+3, M.V.I.-12). It contains nine water-soluble vitamins and three fat-soluble vitamins.

Blood and Blood Cellular Products

Whole blood, citrated. Whole blood contains cellular components (RBC, WBC, and platelets) as well as plasma and its constituents (albumin, globulins, clotting factors, and electrolytes). Whole blood provides complete correction of blood loss by supplying both plasma and cellular components in the correct proportions. It also provides the red blood cells needed to support oxygenation until the patient's own body is able to produce replacement cells. Whole blood must be crossmatched with the recipient's blood type to avoid a transfusion reaction (hemolysis of RBC due to incompatibility of blood types).

Citrated refers to the anticoagulant (citrate) which is commonly used to preserve whole blood and prolong its refrigerated shelf life to 35 days.

DID YOU KNOW? A unit of whole blood contains 500 ml. The common phrase "donate a pint of blood" is fairly accurate and easy for laypersons to remember. One pint is equivalent to 473.17 ml, or nearly one unit of blood.

Packed red blood cells (PRBC). Packed red blood cells is a concentrated preparation of red blood cells (it also contains white blood cells and platelets) with most of the plasma removed. It lacks plasma proteins and clotting factors. Packed red blood cells have an advantage over whole blood in that they can be given without causing fluid overload. This is of special importance in patients with congestive heart failure and in premature infants who need the benefits of whole blood but cannot tolerate the increased blood volume. Packed red blood cells must be crossmatched.

Platelets. Platelets may be administered alone. They are extracted from whole blood and suspended in a small amount of plasma.

Platelets are crossmatched for best results, but in an emergency (and because platelets have a shelf life of only five days and supplies are limited) unmatched platelets may be given. Unmatched platelets do not provoke a transfusion reaction, but the body's antibodies quickly destroy them and they are less effective therapeutically than matched platelets.

Plasma and Plasma Volume Expanders

Plasma and plasma volume expanders are given intravenously to restore blood volume to normal, but they do not contain the cellular components of whole blood and cannot be used to raise the patient's hematocrit or contribute to the oxygen-carrying capacity of the blood. Plasma is derived from human whole blood that has undergone plasmapheresis to remove the cellular components. Plasma volume expanders are manufactured from complex carbohydrates and normal saline; they do not need to be refrigerated and retain their potency for many months.

Fresh frozen plasma (FFP). This consists of human plasma containing all of the plasma proteins and clotting factors. It is frozen to prolong shelf life and then thawed to room temperature before being administered intravenously.

Plasma protein fraction (PPF). Plasma protein fraction is derived from human plasma. It contains 5% plasma proteins mixed with normal saline. It contains no clotting factors. Brand names include:
  Plasmanate
  Plasma-Plex
  Plasmatein

Albumin. This solution, derived from human plasma, contains only the plasma protein albumin, and has no clotting factors. It is prepared in 5% and 25% solutions; the 5% solution approximates the concentration of normal blood plasma. Trade names include:
  Albuminar-5
  Albuminar-25
  Albutein 5%
  Albutein 25%
  Buminate 5%
  Buminate 25%
  Plasbumin-5
  Plasbumin-25

Cryoprecipitate. A plasma extract prepared by freezing and then slowly thawing plasma. It contains concentrated amounts of factor VIII, von Willebrand factor, and fibrinogen.

Dextran. Dextran is a manufactured plasma volume expander consisting of complex carbohydrates with repeating three-dimensional structural units. Normal saline is able to enter these three-dimensional structures to form a viscous fluid that can be used as a substitute for plasma. Dextran is available in three different preparations based on molecular weight.
  dextran 40 (Gentran 40, Rheomacrodex)
  dextran 70 (Macrodex)
  dextran 75 (Gentran 75)

DID YOU KNOW? The combination of the bacteria *Streptococcus mutans* (present in the mouth) and sucrose (table sugar) produces dextran. This somewhat viscous and sticky substance then absorbs the lactic acid produced by other bacteria in the mouth and holds it in contact with the teeth, producing tooth decay.

Hetastarch (Hespan). Hetastarch is a manufactured plasma volume expander derived from a waxy starch commonly found in potatoes, wheat, and corn. Mixed with normal saline, this starch forms a solution similar in viscosity to normal plasma.

Abbreviations in the Glossary

Analges	Analgesia
Anes	Anesthetic
Antibio	Antibiotic
Antifung	Antifungal
Antivir	Antiviral
Cardio	Cardiology
Chemo	Chemotherapy
Derm	Dermatology
Endo	Endocrinology
ENT	Ear, Nose, and Throat (Otorhinolaryngology)
GI	Gastrointestinal
Hem	Hematology
Neuro	Neurology
Ob/Gyn	Obstetrics/Gynecology
Oph	Ophthalmology
Ortho	Orthopedics
Psych	Psychiatric
Resp	Respiratory
Sed/Hyp	Sedative/Hypnotic
Uro	Urology

Note: Page numbers in the Glossary/Index are listed for entries referred to in the text. Entries without page numbers appear only in the Glossary.

Glossary and Index

A, a

A and D (Derm). Topical ointment containing vitamins A and D. 55

Abbokinase (Cardio, Hem). Thrombolytic enzyme. 92

abbreviations, dosage frequency. 47

abbreviations, routes of administration. 21-27

absorption of drug. 28-29

a.c. (before meals).

Accutane (Derm). Oral drug for acne. 5, 52

ACE (angiotensin converting enzyme) **inhibitor** (Cardio). Class of drugs used for hypertension. 82

acebutolol (Sectral) (Cardio). Cardioselective beta blocker drug used for hypertension and arrhythmias. 79, 80

acecainide (Napa) (Cardio). Investigational antiarrhythmic drug. 79

acemannan (Carrisyn) (Antivir). AIDS drug. 146

acetaminophen (Anacin-3, Datril, Liquiprin, Panadol, Tempra) (Analges). Non-aspirin analgesic drugs. 70, 136-137, 139

acetaminophen overdose. 139

acetazolamide (Diamox) (Neuro). Anticonvulsant for absence seizures. 121

acetohexamide (Dymelor) (Endo). Oral antidiabetic drug. 110

acetophenazine (Tindal) (Psych). Phenothiazine antipsychotic drug. 129

acetylcarbromal (Paxarel) (Sed/Hyp). Nonbarbiturate daytime sedative.

acetylcholine (Miochol) (Oph). Miotic drug for glaucoma. 104

acetylcholine (neurotransmitter). 36, 38, 64, 66, 79, 104, 123

acetylcysteine (Mucomyst) (Resp). Mucus-thinning drug; antidote for acetaminophen overdose. 96-97, 139

acetylsalicylic acid (ASA) (Analges). Aspirin. 135

Achromycin (Oph, Derm). Topical tetracycline-type antibiotic. 53, 103, 117, 144

Acidulin (GI). Gastric acid replacement. 68

Achromycin V (Ob/Gyn). Oral tetracycline-type antibiotic. 111

acne, drugs for. 51-52

Actifed (ENT). Decongestant and antihistamine combination. 100

Actigall (GI). Used to dissolve gallstones. 68

actinomycin D (Chemo). Antibiotic used only for chemotherapy. 67

Activase (Cardio, Hem). Thrombolytic enzyme. 92

acyclovir (Zovirax) (Antivir). For herpes simplex virus infection. 54, 117, 148

A.D. (right ear), 25

Adalat (Cardio). Calcium channel blocking drug for angina and hypertension. 78, 82

Adapin (Psych). Tricyclic antidepressant with antianxiety effect. 128, 131

addiction, addictive drugs, 10, 38. See also *Schedule drugs.*

Addison disease, drugs for. 108

Adenocard (Cardio). Antiarrhythmic drug. 79

adenosine (Adenocard) (Cardio). Antiarrhythmic drug. 79

adjuvant therapy. 151
ad lib. (as needed).
administration, drug. See *routes of administration.*
adrenal gland drugs. 108
Adrenalin (Anes). Used with local anesthesia. 158
Adrenalin (Cardio, Resp). Cardiac stimulant and bronchodilator. 27, 88, 89, 95
adrenergic receptor. See *receptor.* 36, 38, 83
Adriamycin (Chemo). Antibiotic used only for chemotherapy. 67, 153
Adrucil (Chemo). Pyrimidine antagonist chemotherapy drug. 151
Adsorbonac (Oph). Topical drug to reduce corneal edema. 105
Advil (Analges, Ob/Gyn, Ortho). Nonsteroidal anti-inflammatory drug. 70, 138
AeroBid (Resp). Inhaled corticosteroid. 95
affective disorders, drugs for. 129-132
Afrin (ENT). Decongestant. 22, 98
Afrinol (ENT). Decongestant. 98
afterload (Cardio). 76
AgNO₃ (Derm). See *silver nitrate.* 55
agonist. 36
AIDS, drugs for. 146-148
AIDS vaccine. 147
Akineton (Neuro). Used to treat Parkinson disease. 123
Albamycin (Antibio). Monobactam antibiotic. 145
albumin. 29-31, 165
Albuminar-5 (Hem). Intravenous albumin 5% to increase blood volume. 165
Albuminar-25 (Hem). Intravenous albumin 25% to increase blood volume. 165
Albutein 5% (Hem). Intravenous albumin 5% to increase blood volume. 165
Albutein 25% (Hem). Intravenous albumin 25% to increase blood volume. 165
albuterol (Proventil, Ventolin) (Resp). Bronchodilator. 94
Aldactazide (Uro). Potassium-wasting and potassium-sparing combination diuretic. 58
Aldactone (Uro). Potassium-sparing diuretic. 58

Aldomet (Cardio). Antihypertensive drug. 83
Aldoril (Cardio). Antihypertensive and diuretic. 84
Alfenta (Anes). I.V. general anesthetic drug. 160
alfentanil (Alfenta) (Anes). I.V. general anesthetic drug. 160
Alferon N (Chemo., Derm., Gyn). Chemotherapy drug. Also given intradermally for genital warts. 54, 117, 155
Alka-Seltzer (GI). Antacid. 62, 90
Alkeran (Chemo). Alkylating chemotherapy drug. 152
alkylating agent (Chemo). Class of chemotherapy drugs. 152
Allerest (ENT). Decongestant and antihistamine combination. 100
allergic drug effect. 35
allergy shots. 26
allopurinol (Zyloprim) (Ortho). Used for gout. 72
alpha-chymotrypsin (Oph). See chymotrypsin. 106
alprazolam (Xanax) (Psych). Benzodiazepine-type antianxiety drug. 127
alprostadil (Prostin VR) (Cardio). Used to keep open ductus arteriosus in newborns with congenital heart disease. 86, 115
Alredase (Oph). Used for diabetic retinopathy. 106
alteplase (Activase) (Cardio, Hem). Thrombolytic enzyme. 92
Alternagel (GI). Antacid. 61
Alupent (Resp). Bronchodilator. 28, 94, 95
Alurate (Sed/Hyp). Barbiturate hypnotic drug. 124
amantadine (Symmetrel) (Neuro, Antivir). Used for Parkinson disease and for influenza virus A. 122, 148
Amcill (Antibio). Penicillin-type antibiotic. 19, 116, 141
amcinonide (Cyclocort) (Derm). Topical corticosteroid anti-inflammatory drug. 53
amdinocillin (Coactin) (Antibio). Penicillin-type antibiotic. 141
amenorrhea, drugs for. 114
Americaine (Derm). Topical anesthetic drug. 158

Amidate (Anes). I.V. drug for induction of general anesthesia. 159

amikacin (Amikin) (Antibio). Aminoglycoside antibiotic. 144

Amikin (Antibio). Aminoglycoside antibiotic. 144

amiloride (Midamor) (Uro). Potassium-sparing diuretic. 58

aminoglycosides (Antibio). Class of antibiotic drugs. 144

aminophylline (Somophyllin) (Resp). Bronchodilator. 94-95

amiodarone (Cordarone) (Cardio). Antiarrhythmic drug. 79

amitriptyline (Elavil, Endep) (Psych). Tricyclic antidepressant. 131

amoxapine (Asendin) (Psych). Tricyclic antidepressant. 131

amoxicillin (Amoxil, Larotid) (Antibio). Penicillin-type antibiotic. 116, 141

Amoxil (Antibio). Penicillin-type antibiotic. 116, 141

amphetamine (Neuro). Used for attention deficit disorder; a CNS stimulant. 124-126

amphetamines (Neuro). Class of CNS stimulants. 130

Amphojel (GI). Antacid. 61

amphotericin B (Fungizone) (Antifung). Oral antifungal/antiyeast drug. 149

ampicillin (Amcill, Omnipen) (Antibio). Penicillin-type antibiotic. 15, 19, 22, 35, 116, 141

ampligen (Antivir). AIDS drug. 146

ampule. 38

amrinone (Inocor) (Cardio). Non-digitalis agent for congestive heart failure. 75

Amvisc (Oph). Aqueous humor replacement. 106

Anacin (Ortho). Over-the-counter nonsteroidal anti-inflammatory drug. 69, 137

Anacin-3 (Analges). Nonaspirin pain reliever. 137

Anafranil (Psych). Tricyclic antidepressant for obsessive-compulsive disorder. 132

analgesics. Class of drugs to relieve pain. 39

analogue. 39

anaphylactic shock. 35

anaphylaxis. 35

Anaprox (Ortho). Nonsteroidal anti-inflammatory drug. 70, 138

Anaspaz (GI). Antispasmodic drug. 59, 64

Anbesol (ENT). Topical anesthetic for mouth. 102

Ancef (Antibio). First-generation cephalosporin antibiotic. 143

Ancobon (Antifung). Systemic antifungal/antiyeast drug. 149

Anectine (Anes). Intraoperative muscle-paralyzing drug. 160

anesthesia, drugs for. 156-161
epidural, 159
general, 24, 39, 158
inhalation, 160
intravenous, 160
local, 39, 72, 158
nerve block, 158
topical, 39, 104, 158
spinal, 27, 159

anesthetics (Anes). Class of drugs used to completely block the sensation of pain. 156-161

angina pectoris, drugs for. 76-78

angiotensin converting enzyme (ACE) inhibitors (Cardio). Class of drugs used for hypertension. 82

anisindione (Miradon) (Hem). Anticoagulant. 92

anisotropine (Valpin) (GI). Antispasmodic drug. 64

anistreplase (APSAC, Eminase) (Cardio, Hem). Thrombolytic enzyme. 92

Ansaid (Ortho). Nonsteroidal anti-inflammatory. 70, 138

ansamycin (Rifabutin) (Antivir). AIDS drug. 146

Anspor (Antibio). First-generation cephalosporin antibiotic. 143

Antabuse (Psych). Used to deter alcohol consumption. 132

antacids (GI). Class of drugs used to neutralize GI acid. 37, 61-62

antagonism, drug. 37

antagonist. 36

antiadrenergic drugs (Cardio). Class of drugs used to treat hypertension. 83

antianginal drugs (Cardio). Class of drugs used to treat or prevent angina pectoris. 76-78

antianxiety drugs (Psych). Class of drugs for neurosis/anxiety; known as minor tranquilizers and anxiolytic drugs. 126-128

antiarrhythmia, drugs for. 78-80

antibiotics (Antibio). Class of drugs used to inhibit the growth of or kill bacteria, particularly pathogens. 39, 59, 101, 103, 141-145

antibiotics
broad-spectrum
chemotherapy (Chemo). 152-153
topical. 53
urinary tract. See *anti-infectives.*

anticoagulant drugs (Hem). Class of drugs used to inhibit blood clotting. 92

anticholinergic. Class of drugs which oppose the action of acetylcholine. 39, 63-64

antidepressants (Psych). Class of drugs for depression. 33, 39, 129-131

antidiabetics (Endo). Class of drugs given orally for diabetes. 109-110

antidiarrheals (GI). Class of drugs to treat diarrhea. 64

antiemetic (GI). Class of drugs to relieve nausea and vomiting. 39, 66-67, 154

antihistamines (ENT). Class of drugs to block effects of histamine released in allergic reactions. 6, 29, 33, 37, 39, 63, 99, 124

antihypertensives (Cardio). Class of drugs used to treat high blood pressure. 39, 80-82

anti-infectives, urinary tract (Uro). 59, 140

anti-inflammatory drugs (Derm, Ortho). Class of drugs used to decrease inflammation. 39

antimetabolites (Chemo). Class of chemotherapy drugs. 151-152

antineoplastic drugs. Class of chemotherapy drugs. 39

antipruritics (Derm). Class of drugs to relieve itching. 39, 54-55

antipsychotic drugs (Psych). Class of drugs for psychosis; also known as major tranquilizers. 128-129

antiseptic. 39

antispasmodics (GI, Ortho, Uro). Class of drugs used to stop muscle spasm. 39, 59, 63-64.

antituberculosis drugs (Resp). Class of drugs used to treat tuberculosis. 96

antitussives (ENT). Class of drugs to suppress dry, nonproductive cough. 39, 99

Antivert (GI). Used for vertigo. 67

antiviral. Class of drugs to treat viral infections. 39, 54, 146-148

Anturane (Ortho). Used for gout. 72

anxiolytic drugs (Psych). Class of drugs for neurosis/anxiety. 126-128

A.P.L. (Ob/Gyn). Ovulation-stimulating agent for infertility. 111

apothecary system. 44, 46

apraclonidine (Iopidine) (Oph). Miotic drug for glaucoma. 105, 124

Apresazide (Cardio). Antihypertensive and diuretic. 84

Apresoline (Cardio). Vasodilator. 14, 83

aprobarbital (Alurate) (Sed/Hyp). Barbiturate hypnotic drug. 124

APSAC (Cardio, Hem). Abbreviation for anistreplase. Thrombolytic enzyme. 92

AquaMEPHYTON (Hem). Used to reverse oral anticoagulant overdose; also given prophylactically to prevent bleeding. 93

aqueous, 23

Aramine (Anes). Used to treat hypotension from spinal anesthesia. 161

Ara-A (Antivir). Used for herpes simplex virus infection. 148

Ara-C (Chemo). Pyrimidine antagonist chemotherapy drug. 151

Aristocort (Derm, Endo, Ortho). Topical and oral corticosteroid anti-inflammatory drug. 46, 53, 71, 108

Aristospan (Ortho). Oral corticosteroid anti-inflammatory drug. 71

Arlidin (Cardio). Peripheral vasodilating drug. 84

arrhythmias, drugs for. 6, 10, 19, 24, 78-80

Artane (Neuro). Used to treat Parkinson disease. 123

arthritis, drugs for. 69, 71

Arthropan (Ortho). Over-the-counter non-steroidal anti-inflammatory drug. 69, 136

A.S. (left ear). 25

ASA (Analges). Aspirin. 135

A.S.A. Enseals (Ortho). Over-the-counter nonsteroidal anti-inflammatory drug. 69, 136

Ascriptin A/D (Ortho). Over-the-counter nonsteroidal anti-inflammatory drug. 69, 136

Asendin (Psych). Tricyclic antidepressant. 14, 15, 131

asparaginase (Elspar) (Chemo). Chemotherapy drug. 154

aspirin (Cardio, Hem). Used to prevent second heart attack; anticoagulant. 78, 92

aspirin (Analges). Nonsteroidal anti-inflammatory drug; pain reliever. 5, 6, 9, 33, 61, 63, 69, 70, 78, 92, 135, 136, 138

astemizole (Hismanal) (ENT). Antihistamine. 99

Atarax (Derm). Antianxiety agent given for severe itching. 55

atenolol (Tenormin) (Cardio, Analges). Cardioselective beta blocker drug, used for angina and hypertension; also used for migraine headaches. 77, 79-80, 138

Ativan (Psych). Benzodiazepine-type anti-anxiety drug. 13, 127

atracurium besylate (Tracium) (Anes). Intraoperative muscle-paralyzing agent. 160

Atromid-S (Cardio). Used to lower hyper-triglyceridemia. 21, 85

atropine (Anes, Cardio). Facilitates endotracheal intubation by decreasing secretions; antiarrhythmic drug. 79, 88, 90, 160

atropine (Oph). Mydriatic drug. 3-5, 105

Atrovent (Resp). Bronchodilator. 94

attention deficit disorder, drugs for. 124

A.U. (both ears).

Augmentin (Antibio). Combination of amoxicillin and beta lactamase inhibitor to kill resistant bacteria. 144

Auralgan Otic (ENT). Topical anesthetic for ear. 102

auranofin (Ridaura). (Ortho). Gold salts used for arthritis. 71

Aureomycin (Oph). Topical antibiotic for eye. 103

aurothioglucose (Solganal). (Ortho). Gold salts used for arthritis. 71

AVC (Ob/Gyn). Topical sulfa drug for vaginal yeast infections. 115

Aveeno (Derm). Topical antipruritic bath. 55

Aventyl (Psych). Tricyclic antidepressant. 131

Axid (GI). H_2 blocker to heal ulcers. 62

Aygestin (OB/GYN). Used to treat amenorrhea. 114

Azactam (Antibio). Monobactam antibiotic. 145

azidothymidine (AZT). (Antivir). AIDS drug. 146-147

Azlin (Antibio). Penicillin-type antibiotic. 141

azlocillin (Azlin). (Antibio). Penicillin-type antibiotic. 141

Azmacort (Resp). Inhaled corticosteroid. 14, 95

Azo Gantrisin (Uro). Sulfonamide anti-infective and urinary tract analgesic combination drug. 59

AZT (Antivir). AIDS drug. 146-147

aztreonam (Azactam). (Antibio). Monobactam antibiotic. 145

Azulfidine (Antibio). Sulfonamide anti-infective for ulcerative colitis. 66, 140

B, b

baby, see *pediatric patients.*

bacampicillin (Spectrobid) (Antibio). Penicillin-type antibiotic. 116, 141

bacitracin (Derm, Oph). Topical and ophthalmic antibiotic. 53, 103

baclofen (Lioresal) (Ortho). Used for severe muscle spasticity. 72

bacteria
gram-negative. 144.
gram-positive. 144

bactericidal. Class of drugs to kill bacteria. 39

bacteriostatic. Class of drugs to inhibit the growth of bacteria. 39

Bactine (Derm). Topical over-the-counter antibiotic combination. 53

Bactocill (Antibio). Penicillin-type antibiotic. 141

Bactrim (Antibio). Combination antibiotic and sulfonamide anti-infective. 144

Bactrim DS (Antibio.). Double strength Bactrim. 14, 144

baking soda (GI). Antacid. 62

balanced salt solution (BSS) (Oph). Intraocular irrigant/protectant. 106

Balnetar (Derm). Coal tar solution for psoriasis. 52

barbiturate (Sed/Hyp). Class of drugs used to produce sedation and sleep; also used for epilepsy. 120, 123-124

barbiturate, ultrashort-acting (Anes). Used to induce general anesthesia. 159

Basaljel (GI). Antacid. 61

Bayer (Ortho). Over-the-counter nonsteroidal anti-inflammatory drug. 69, 136

Baypress (Cardio). Investigational calcium channel blocking drug. 82

beclomethasone (Beclovent, Vanceril) (Resp). Inhaled corticosteroid. 95

beclomethasone (Beconase, Vancenase) (ENT) Intranasal corticosteroid.

Beclovent (Resp). Inhaled corticosteroid. 95

Beconase (ENT). Intranasal corticosteroid. 101

beef pancreas. 5

belladonna plant. 3, 5, 105

Bellergal-S (GI). Antispasmodic and sedative combination drug. 64

Benadryl (Derm). Topical antihistamine, antipruritic. 22, 32, 54

Benadryl (ENT, GI). Antihistamine; used for motion sickness. 6, 32, 66, 99

bendroflumethiazide (Naturetin) (Uro). Thiazide diuretic. 57

Benemid (Ortho). Used for gout. 72

Bentyl (GI). Antispasmodic. 64

Benylin (ENT). Decongestant and antihistamine combination. 99, 100

Benzamycin (Derm). Erythromycin/benzoyl peroxide combination for acne. 51

benzocaine (Americaine, Dermoplast) (Derm). Topical anesthetic. 158

benzocaine (Auralgan Otic) (ENT). Topical anesthetic for ear. 102

benzodiazepines (Psych). Class of drugs used to treat anxiety and insomnia. 13, 15, 123-124, 127-128

benzoyl peroxide (Derm). Topical antibiotic for acne. 51

benzquinamide (Emete-Con) (GI). Antiemetic. 66

benztropine mesylate (Cogentin) (Neuro). Used for Parkinson disease. 123

Berotec (Resp). An investigational bronchodilator. 94

beta blockers (Cardio, Analges). Class of drugs for angina, arrhythmias, hypertension; migraine headaches. 6, 79-81

beta blockers
cardioselective (Cardio). 81
nonselective (Cardio). 80
selective (Cardio). 81

Betadine (Derm). Topical antibiotic soap and solution. 55

Betagan (Oph). Beta blocking drug for glaucoma. 105

beta-lactam ring. 141

beta-lactamase. 141

betamethasone (Celestone) (Endo, Ortho). Oral corticosteroid anti-inflammatory drug. 71, 108

bupivacaine (Marcaine). (Oph, Ortho). Local anesthetic given by retrobulbar injection; given by intra-articular injection. 72, 106

buprenorphine (Buprenex). (Analges). Narcotic analgesic drug. 135

Buprenex (Analges). Narcotic analgesic drug. 135

bupropion (Wellbutrin). (Psych). Antidepressant. 131

Burow's solution (Derm). Topical antipruritic solution. 55

BuSpar (Psych). Antianxiety drug. 128

buspirone (BuSpar). (Psych). Antianxiety drug. 128

busulfan (Myleran). (Chemo). Chemotherapy drug. 152

butabarbital (Butisol). (Sed/Hyp). Barbiturate hypnotic drug. 124

Butazolidin (Ortho). Anti-inflammatory drug. 71-72

Butisol (Sed/Hyp). Barbiturate hypnotic drug. 124

butoconazole (Femstat). (Ob/Gyn). Topical vaginal antiyeast drug. 115

butorphanol (Stadol). (Analges). Nonnarcotic analgesic drug. 135

butterfly needle. 42

■

C, c

c̄ *(cum)*, with

Cafergot (Analges). Used for migraine headaches. 139

Caladryl (Derm). Topical antihistamine and antipruritic combination drug. 54

calamine (Derm). Topical antipruritic drug. 22, 54-55

Calan (Cardio, Analges). Calcium channel blocker drug for angina, arrhythmias, and hypertension; also for migraine headaches. 78-79, 82, 139

Calcimar (Ortho). Calcium supplement for osteoporosis. 72

Calciparine (Hem). Anticoagulant. 92

calcitonin (Calcimar). (Ortho). Calcium supplement for osteoporosis. 72

calcitriol (Rocaltrol). (Ortho). Increases bone absorption of calcium. 72

calcium channel blockers (Cardio, Analges). Class of drugs for angina and hypertension; migraine headaches. 6, 77-78, 81-82

calcium chloride (Emerg). Cardiac stimulant. 90

CaldeCort (Derm). Topical corticosteroid anti-inflammatory drug. 53

Cama (Ortho). Nonsteroidal anti-inflammatory drug. 69, 136

Candida albicans. 101-102, 115, 146, 148-149

candidiasis. 102, 148

cannabinoid (GI). Active ingredient in marijuana; antiemetic. 67

caplet. 21-22

Capoten (Cardio). ACE inhibitor drug used for hypertension. 82

Capozide (Cardio). Antihypertensive and diuretic. 84

capsaicin (Zostrix). (Derm). Topical drug for herpes zoster infection. 54

capsule. 21-23

captopril (Capoten). (Cardio). ACE inhibitor drug used for hypertension. 82

Carafate (GI). Antiulcer drug. 28, 63

carbachol (Miostat). (Oph). Miotic drug for glaucoma. 104

carbamazepine (Tegretol). (Neuro). Used to treat tonic-clonic seizures. 121

carbenicillin (Geopen, Pyopen). (Antibio). Penicillin-type antibiotic. 116, 141

carbidopa (Lodosyn). (Neuro). Used to treat Parkinson disease. 122

Carbocaine (Anes). Local/regional anesthetic. 158-159

carboplatin (Paraplatin). (Chemo). Chemotherapy drug. 152

carboprost (Hemabate). (Ob/Gyn). Prostaglandin used to abort fetus.

Cardene (Cardio). Calcium channel blocker drug used for angina and hypertension. 78, 82

cardiac glycosides (Cardio). Class of digitalis drugs used for congestive heart failure. 74-75

Cardilate (Cardio). Antianginal drug. 77

Cardioquin (Cardio). Antiarrhythmic drug. 79

cardioselective beta blockers. 81

Cardizem (Cardio). Calcium channel blocker used for angina and hypertension. 78, 82

Cardura (Cardio). An alpha₁ blocker drug used for hypertension. 83

carisoprodol (Soma) (Ortho). Skeletal muscle relaxant. 72

carmustine (BiCNU) (Chemo). Alkylating chemotherapy agent. 152

carprofen (Rimadyl) (Ortho). Investigational nonsteroidal anti-inflammatory drug. 70, 138

Carrisyn (Antivir). AIDS drug. 146

carteolol (Cartrol). (Cardio). Nonselective beta blocker drug used for hypertension. 80

Cartrol (Cardio). Nonselective beta blocker drug used for hypertension. 80

cascara (GI). Laxative. 65

Catapres (Cardio). Antihypertensive drug. 83

Catarase (Oph). Used to free lens in intraocular surgery. 106

catheter, umbilical artery/vein. 27

cc (cubic centimeter).

Ceclor (Antibio). Cephalosporin antibiotic. 35, 143

Cedilanid-D (Cardio). Digitalis drug for congestive heart failure. 75

CeeNu (Chemo). Alkylating chemotherapy drug. 152

cefaclor (Ceclor) (Antibio). Cephalosporin antibiotic. 143

cefadroxil (Duricef, Ultracef). (Antibio). Cephalosporin antibiotic. 143

Cefadyl (Antibio). First-generation cephalosporin antibiotic. 143

cefamandole (Mandol) (Antibio). Cephalosporin antibiotic. 143

cefazolin (Ancef, Kefzol) (Antibio). First-generation cephalosporin antibiotic. 143

cefixime (Suprax) (Antibio). Third-generation cephalosporin antibiotic. 143

Cefizox (Antibio). Third-generation cephalosporin antibiotic. 143

cefmetazole (Zefazone) (Antibio). Second-general cephalosporin antibiotic. 143

Cefobid (Antibio). Third-generation cephalosporin antibiotic. 116, 143

cefonicid (Monocid) (Antibio). Second-generation cephalosporin antibiotic. 143

cefoperazone (Cefobid) (Antibio). Third-generation cephalosporin antibiotic. 116, 143

ceforanide (Precef). (Antibio). Second-generation cephalosporin antibiotic. 116, 143

Cefotan (Antibio). Second-generation cephalosporin antibiotic. 116, 143

cefotaxime (Claforan) (Antibio). Third-generation cephalosporin antibiotic. 116, 143

cefotetan (Cefotan) (Antibio). Second-generation cephalosporin antibiotic. 116, 143

cefoxitin (Mefoxin) (Antibio). Second-generation cephalosporin antibiotic. 116, 143

ceftazidime (Fortaz, Tazidime) (Antibio). Third-generation cephalosporin antibiotic. 143

Ceftin (Antibio). Second-generation cephalosporin antibiotic. 143

ceftizoxime (Cefizox) (Antibio). Third-generation cephalosporin antibiotic. 143

ceftriaxone (Rocephin) (Antibio). Third-generation cephalosporin antibiotic. 116, 143

cefuroxime (Ceftin, Zinacef) (Antibio). Second-generation cephalosporin antibiotic. 116, 143

Celestone (Endo, Ortho). Corticosteroid anti-inflammatory drug. 71, 108

Celontin (Neuro). For absence seizures. 121

Centrax (Psych). Benzodiazepine-type anti-anxiety drug. 13, 128

Cepacol (ENT). Topical anesthetic for mouth. 21, 102

cephalexin (Keflex, Keftab) (Antibio). First-generation cephalosporin antibiotic. 143

cephalosporin (Antibio). Class of antibacterial drugs. 15, 35, 141-144
    first-generation, 143
    second-generation, 143
    third-generation, 143

cephalothin (Keflin) (Antibio). First-generation cephalosporin antibiotic. 143

cephapirin (Cefadyl) (Antibio). First-generation cephalosporin antibiotic. 143

cephradine (Anspor, Velosef) (Antibio). First-generation cephalosporin antibiotic. 143

Cerubidine (Chemo). Antibiotic used only for chemotherapy. 153

Cerumenex (ENT). Topical wax softener for ear. 102

Cesamet (GI). Used for nausea after chemotherapy. 67

chemical name of drug. 13, 49

chemical structure of drug. 13-14

chemotherapy, drugs for. 33, 48, 67, 150-155

chemotherapy protocols. 154

Chenix (GI). Used to dissolve gallstones. 68

chenodiol (Chenix) (GI). Used to dissolve gallstones. 68

Chlamydia trachomatis. 117

chloral hydrate (Noctec) (Sed/Hyp). Non-barbiturate night-time sedative. 29, 123

chlorambucil (Leukeran) (Chemo). Alkylating chemotherapy drug. 152

chloramphenicol (Chloromycetin, Chloroptic) (Antiobio). Topical ophthalmic and oral antibiotic. 53, 103, 145

Chloraseptic (ENT). Topical anesthetic for mouth. 102

chlordiazepoxide (Librium) (Psych, Neuro). Benzodiazepine-type antianxiety drug; for alcohol withdrawal seizures. 15, 125, 127

chlormezanone (Trancopal) (Psych). Antianxiety drug. 128

chloroform (Anes). 157

Chloromycetin Otic (ENT). Topical ear antibiotic. 101

Chloromycetin (Antibio). Oral, ophthalmic, and topical antibiotic. 53, 103, 145

chloroprocaine (Nesacaine) (Anes). Local/regional anesthetic. 158-159

Chloroptic (Oph). Topical antibiotic. 103

chlorothiazide (Diuril). (Uro). Thiazide diuretic. 57

chlorotrianisene (TACE) (Ob/Gyn). Estrogen replacement for menopause. 114

chlorpheniramine (Chlor-Trimeton) (ENT). Decongestant. 99

chlorpromazine (Thorazine) (Psych, GI). Phenothiazine antipsychotic drug; antiemetic. 66-67, 128-129

chlorpropamide (Diabinese) (Endo). Oral antidiabetic drug. 110

chlorprothixene (Taractan) (Psych). Antipsychotic drug. 129

chlortetracycline (Aureomycin) (Oph). Topical eye antibiotic. 103

chlorthalidone (Hygroton) (Uro). Diuretic. 57

chlorzoxazone (Parafon Forte DSC) (Ortho). Skeletal muscle relaxant. 72

Chlor-Trimeton (ENT). Decongestant. 99

Choledyl (Resp). Bronchodilator. 95

cholestyramine (Cholybar, Questran) (Cardio). Used for hypercholesterolemia. 85

cholinergic receptor. See receptor.

Choloxin (Cardio). Used for hypercholesterolemia. 85

Cholybar (Cardio). Used for hypercholesterolemia. 85

chronotropic effect, negative (Cardio). 74

Chronulac (GI). Laxative. 65

Chymodiactin (Ortho, Neuro). Used to dissolve herniated disk. 73

chymopapain (Chymodiactin) (Ortho, Neuro). Used to dissolve herniated disk. 73

chymotrypsin (Catarase, Zolyse) (Oph). Used to free lens in intraocular surgery. 106

ciclopirox (Loprox) (Derm). Topical antifungal agent. 54

cifenline succinate (Cipralan) (Cardio). Investigative antiarrhythmic drug. 79

cimetidine (Tagamet) (GI). H_2 blocker to heal ulcers. 19, 62-63.

cinchona bark. 5

Cinobac (Uro). Urinary tract antibiotic. 59

cinoxacin (Cinobac) (Uro). Urinary tract antibiotic. 59

Cipralan (Cardio). Investigational antiarrhythmic drug. 79

Cipro (Antibio). Antibiotic. 14, 116, 145

ciprofloxacin (Cipro) (Antibio). Antibiotic. 14, 116, 145

cisplatin (cis-platinum, Platinol) (Chemo). Alkylating chemotherapy drug. 152

cis-platinum (Chemo). Alkylating chemotherapy drug. 152

citrated whole blood (Hem). Whole blood with citrate preservative. 164

Citrucel (GI) Laxative. 65

Claforan (Antibio). Third-generation cephalosporin antibiotic. 116, 143

Claritin (ENT). Investigational decongestant. 99

Clearasil (Derm). Topical acne preparation. 51

clemastine (Tavist) (ENT). Decongestant. 99

Cleocin (Antibio). Antibiotic. 145

Cleocin T (Derm). Topical antibiotic for acne. 51

clidinium (Quarzan) (GI). Antispasmodic drug. 64

clindamycin (Cleocin) (Antibio). Antibiotic. 145

clindamycin (Cleocin T) (Derm). Topical antibiotic for acne. 51

Clinoril (Ortho). Nonsteroidal anti-inflammatory drug. 70, 72, 138

clobazam (Frisium) (Psych). Investigational benzodiazepine-type antianxiety drug. 127

clocortolone (Cloderm) (Derm). Topical corticosteroid anti-inflammatory drug. 53

Cloderm (Derm). Topical corticosteroid anti-inflammatory drug. 53

clofibrate (Atromid-S) (Cardio). Used for hypertriglyceridemia. 85

clomipramine (Anafranil) (Psych). Tricyclic antidepressant for obsessive-compulsive disorder. 132

Clomid (Ob/Gyn) Ovulation-stimulating drug for infertility. 111

clomiphene (Clomid) (Ob/Gyn) Ovulation-stimulating agent for infertility. 111

clonazepam (Klonopin) (Neuro). Used to treat absence seizures. 121

clonidine (Catapres) (Cardio). Antihypertensive agent. 83

clorazepate (Tranxene) (Neuro, Psych). Anticonvulsant; benzodiazepine-type antianxiety drug. 121, 127

clotrimazole (Gyne-Lotrimin) (Ob/Gyn) Topical antiyeast drug for vaginal infection. 115

clotrimazole (Lotrimin, Mycelex) (Derm, ENT, Ob/Gyn). Topical anti-fungal/antiyeast drug. 54, 101

cloxacillin (Cloxapen, Tegopen) (Antibio). Penicillin-type antibiotic. 141

Cloxapen (Antibio). Penicillin-type antibiotic. 141

clozapine (Clozaril) (Psych). Antipsychotic drug for schizophrenia. 132

Clozaril (Psych). Antipsychotic drug for schizophrenia. 132

Coactin (Antibio). Penicillin-type antibiotic. 141

CoAdvil (ENT). Decongestant and pain reliever. 100

coal tar preparations. 52

cocaine (ENT). Topical vasoconstrictor and anesthetic. 102

cocoa butter. 6, 23

codeine (ENT). Narcotic antitussive; analgesic. 10, 33, 99, 135.

Code of Hammurabi. 8

Cogentin (Neuro). Used to treat Parkinson disease. 123

Cognex (Neuro). Investigational drug for Alzheimer disease. 125

Colace (GI). Laxative. 65

colchicine (Ortho). Used for gout. 4, 72

Colchicum autumnale (plant). 4

Colestid (Cardio). Used for hypercholesterolemia. 85

colestipol (Colestid) (Cardio). Used for hypercholesterolemia. 85

colfosceril palmitate (Exosurf, Survanta) (Resp). Investigational lung surfactant supplement for premature infants. 97

colistin (Coly-Mycin S) (Antibio). Antibiotic. 145

Coly-Mycin S Otic (ENT). Topical corticosteroid and antibiotic for ear. 101

Coly-Mycin S (Antibio). Oral antibiotic. 145

CoLyte (GI). Bowel evacuant/bowel prep. 65

Combipres (Cardio). Antihypertensive and diuretic. 84

Compazine (GI). Antiemetic. 66-67

Comprecin (Antibio). Investigational antibiotic. 145

computer-aided drug design. 16

Comtrex (ENT). Decongestant, antihistamine, non-narcotic antitussive, and pain reliever. 100

congestive heart failure, drugs for. 3, 20, 74

conjugated estrogens (Premarin) (Ob/Gyn). Estrogen replacement for menopause. 114

Constant-T (Resp). Bronchodilator. 95

Contac (ENT). Decongestant and antihistamine combination. 100

contraceptive, oral (Ob/Gyn). 112-114

controlled substance. 10-11, 49, 64

Controlled Substance Act. 10, 49

Cordarone (Cardio). Antiarrhythmic drug. 79

Cordran (Derm). Topical corticosteroid anti-inflammatory drug. 53

Cordran-N (Derm). Topical corticosteroid anti-inflammatory/antibiotic. 53

Corgard (Cardio, Analges). Nonselective beta blocker drug used for angina and hypertension; also used for migraine headaches. 77, 79-80, 138

Correctol (GI). Laxative. 65

Cortaid (Derm). Topical corticosteroid anti-inflammatory drug. 53

Cortef (Derm, Endo, Ortho). Topical and oral corticosteroid anti-inflammatory drug. 53, 71, 108

Cortenema (GI). Topical corticosteroid anti-inflammatory drug for ulcerative colitis. 66

corticosteroids Class of anti-inflammatory drugs. 6, 26, 39, 52-53, 66, 71, 95, 100-101, 104, 154

Cortifoam (GI). Topical corticosteroid anti-inflammatory drug for ulcerative colitis. 66

cortisone (Cortone) (Endo, Ortho). Corticosteroid anti-inflammatory drug. 6, 71, 108

Cortisporin Otic (ENT). Topical corticosteroid and antibiotic for ear. 101

Cortisporin (Derm). Topical corticosteroid anti-inflammatory/antibiotic. 53

Cortone (Ortho). Oral corticosteroid anti-inflammatory drug. 71

Cortril (Derm). Topical corticosteroid anti-inflammatory drug. 53

Cosmegen (Chemo). Antibiotic used only for chemotherapy. 67

Cotazym (GI). Digestive enzyme. 68

cough syrup. 10, 22

Coumadin (Hem). Anticoagulant. 92

CR (abbreviation for *controlled release*). 39

crash cart (Emerg). Portable cart holding all emergency resuscitation drugs/devices. 88

crash induction of anesthesia.

creams, topical. 22

cromolyn (Intal) (Resp). Mast cell inhibitor for bronchial asthma. 95-96

cromolyn (Nasalcrom, Opticrom) (ENT, Oph). Topical mast cell inhibitor for allergic rhinitis and allergic ophthalmitis. 102, 106

cromolyn (Gastrocrom) (GI). Oral mast cell inhibitor for food allergies. 68

cryoprecipitate (Hem). Plasma extract with clotting factors. 93, 165

crystalloid. General term for normal saline and lactated Ringer's intravenous fluids. 163

Crystodigin (Cardio). Digitalis drug used for congestive heart failure. 75

cubic centimeter (cc). 45

curare (Anes). 157

cyanide. 8, 21

cyanocobalamin (Cardio). For pernicious anemia, given by I.M. injection. 87

cyclacillin (Cyclapen-W) (Antibio). Penicillin-type antibiotic. 141

Cyclapen-W (Antibio). Penicillin-type antibiotic. 141

cyclobenzaprine (Flexeril) (Ortho). Skeletal muscle relaxant. 72

Cyclocort (Derm). Topical corticosteroid anti-inflammatory drug. 53

Cyclogyl (Oph). Mydriatic drug. 105

cyclopentolate (Cyclogyl) (Oph). Mydriatic drug. 105

cyclophosphamide (Cytoxan) (Chemo). Alkylating chemotherapy drug. 67, 152

cyclopropane (Anes). 157

Cylert (Neuro). For attention deficit disorder, a CNS stimulant. 124

cyproheptadine (Periactin) (Derm). Oral antipruritic drug. 54

cytarabine (Ara-C, Cytosar-U) (Chemo). Pyrimidine antagonist chemotherapy drug. 151

Cytomel (Endo). Thyroid hormone replacement. 107

Cytosar-U (Chemo). Pyrimidine antagonist chemotherapy drug. 151

Cytospaz (Uro). Antispasmodic. 59

Cytotec (GI). Used to prevent ulcers in patients on NSAID therapy. 63, 73, 139

Cytovene (Antivir). Used for cytomegalovirus. 148

Cytoxan (Chemo). Chemotherapy drug. 67, 152

■

D, d

D-50-W. Intravenous fluid of 50% dextrose in water. 163.

D5/LR. Intravenous fluid of dextrose 5% in lactated Ringer's. 163

D5/NS. Intravenous fluid of dextrose 5% in normal saline.

D-5-W. Intravenous fluid of 5% dextrose in water. 163

D-10-W. Intravenous fluid of 10% dextrose in water. 163

dacarbazine (DTIC-Dome) (Chemo). Chemotherapy drug. 67, 154

dactinomycin (actinomycin D, Cosmegen) (Chemo). Antibiotic used only for chemotherapy. 67, 153

Dalgan (Analges). Nonnarcotic analgesic drug. 135

Dalmane (Sed/Hyp). Nonbarbiturate benzodiazepine drug for insomnia. 123

danazol (Danocrine) (Ob/Gyn). Used to treat endometriosis. 112

Danocrine (Ob/Gyn). Used to treat endometriosis. 112

Dantrium (Anes). Used to treat intraoperative malignant hypothermia. 161

Dantrium (Ortho). For severe muscle spasticity. 72

dantrolene (Dantrium) (Anes, Ortho). Used for intraoperative malignant hypothermia; used for severe muscle spasticity. 72, 161

Daricon (GI). Antispasmodic drug. 64

Darvocet-N (Analges). Narcotic analgesic drug. 137

Darvon (Analges). Narcotic analgesic drug. 135

Darvon Compound (Analges). Narcotic analgesic drug. 10, 135

Datril (Analges). Non-narcotic analgesic drug. 137

daunorubicin (Cerubidine) (Chemo). Antibiotic used only for chemotherapy. 153

DDAVP (Endo). Used to treat diabetes insipidus, enuresis. 108

ddC (Antivir). AIDS drug. 146

ddI (Antivir). AIDS drug. 146

DEA (Drug Enforcement Administration).

Decabid (Cardio). Investigational antiarrhythmic drug. 79

Decaderm (Derm). Topical corticosteroid anti-inflammatory drug. 53

Decadron (Derm, Endo, Oph, Ortho). Topical and oral corticosteroid anti-inflammatory drug. 53, 71, 104, 108

Decadron Respihaler (Pulm). Inhaled corticosteroid anti-inflammatory drug. 95

Decadron Turbinaire (ENT). Intranasal corticosteroid.

Decholin (GI). Decreases bile thickness. 68

Declomycin (Antibio). Tetracycline-type antibiotic. 116-117, 144

Deconamine (ENT). Decongestant and antihistamine combination. 100

decongestants (ENT). Class of drugs which act as vasoconstrictors on mucous membranes. 40, 98

dehydrocholic acid (Decholin) (GI). Decreases bile thickness. 68

Deltasone (Endo, Ortho). Oral corticosteroid anti-inflammatory drug. 71, 108

Delta-Cortef (Endo, Ortho). Oral corticosteroid anti-inflammatory drug. 71, 108

demecarium (Humorsol) (Oph). Miotic drug for glaucoma. 105

demeclocycline (Declomycin) (Antibio). Tetracycline-type antibiotic. 116-117, 144

Demerol (Anes). Preoperative drug to sedate, relieve pain. 10, 26, 135, 161

Demulen 1/35 (Ob/Gyn). Combination progesterone/estrogen oral contraceptive. 113

Demulen 1/50 (Ob/Gyn). Combination progesterone/estrogen oral contraceptive. 113

Denorex (Derm). Coal tar shampoo for psoriasis. 52

Depakene (Neuro). Used to treat absence seizures. 121

Depakote (Neuro). Used to treat absence seizures. 121

dependence, physical/psychological. 10

Depogen (Ob/Gyn). Estrogen replacement for menopause. 114

Depo-Estradiol (Ob/Gyn). Estrogen replacement for menopause. 114

Depo-Medrol (Endo, Ortho). Oral corticosteroid anti-inflammatory drug. 71, 108

Depo-Provera (Chemo). Hormonal chemotherapy drug. 153

depression, drugs for. 129-132

Deprol (Psych). Combination antianxiety drug and antidepressant. 132

dermatology, drugs for. 51-56

Dermoplast (Derm). Topical anesthetic drug. 158

Desenex (Derm). Topical antifungal drug. 54

deserpidine (Harmonyl) (Cardio). Antihypertensive drug. 83

desiccated thyroid (Endo). Thyroid hormone replacement. 107

designing drugs. 15-17

desipramine (Norpramin) (Psych). Tricyclic antidepressant. 131

Desitin (Derm). Topical drug with zinc and vitamin A. 55

deslanoside (Cedilanid-D) (Cardio). Digitalis agent for congestive heart failure. 75

desmopressin (DDAVP) (Endo). Used for diabetes insipidus, enuresis. 108

desonide (Tridesilon) (Derm). Topical corticosteroid anti-inflammatory drug. 53

desoximetasone (Topicort) (Derm). Topical corticosteroid anti-inflammatory drug. 53

desoxycorticosterone (Percorten) (Endo). Used to treat Addison disease. 108

Desoxyn (Neuro). For attention deficit disorder, a CNS stimulant. 124

Desyrel (Psych). Antidepressant. 131

dexamethasone (Decadron, Maxidex) (Oph). Topical corticosteroid. 104

dexamethasone (Decadron Respihaler) (Resp). Corticosteroid. 95

dexamethasone (Decaderm, Decadron) (Derm). Topical corticosteroid. 53

dexamethasone (Decadron Turbinaire) (ENT). Intranasal corticosteroid. 101

dexamethasone (Decadron) (Endo, Ortho). Oral corticosteroid anti-inflammatory drug. 71

Dexedrine (Neuro). Used for attention deficit disorder, a CNS stimulant. 124

dexpanthenol (Ilopan) (GI). Gastric stimulant. 66

dextran 40 (Gentran 40, Rheomacrodex) (Hem). Plasma volume expander. 165

dextran 70 (Macrodex) (Hem). Plasma volume expander. 165

dextran 75 (Gentran 75) (Hem). Plasma volume expander. 165

dextran sulfate (Uendex) (Antivir). AIDS drug. 146

dextroamphetamine (Dexedrine) (Neuro). Used for attention deficit disorder, a CNS stimulant. 124

dextromethorphan (Sucrets, Pertussin) (ENT). Non-narcotic antitussive drug. 99

dextrorotary. 40

dextrose 10% in water (D-10-W). Intravenous fluid. 163

dextrose 50% in water (D-50-W). Intravenous fluid. 163

dextrose 5% in lactated Ringer's (D5/LR). Intravenous fluid. 163

dextrose 5% in normal saline (D5/NS). Intravenous fluid. 163

dextrose 5% in water (D-5-W). Intravenous fluid. 163

dextrothyroxine (Choloxin). (Cardio). Used to treat hypercholesterolemia. 85

dezocine (Dalgan) (Analges). Non-narcotic analgesic drug. 135

D.H.E. 45 (Analges). Used for migraine headaches. 138

DiaBeta (Endo). Oral antidiabetic drug. 110

diabetes mellitus, drugs for. 109-110.

Diabinese (Endo). Oral antidiabetic drug. 110

Diamox (Neuro). Used to treat absence seizures. 121

Diapid (Endo). Used to treat diabetes insipidus. 108

diazepam (Valium) (Anes). Preoperative drug to decrease anxiety. 160

diazepam (Valium) (Neuro, Ortho). Used for status epilepticus; skeletal muscle relaxer. 72, 125

diazepam (Valium) (Psych). Benzodiazepine-type antianxiety drug. 13, 15, 127

diazoxide (Hyperstat) (Cardio). Used for hypertensive crisis. 82

dibucaine (Nupercainal) (Derm). Topical anesthetic drug. 158

diclofenac (Voltaren) (Ortho). Nonsteroidal anti-inflammatory drug. 70, 138

dicloxacillin (Dynapen, Pathocil) (Antibio). Penicillin-type antibiotic. 141

dicumarol (Hem). Anticoagulant. 92

dicyclomine (Bentyl, Di-Spaz) (GI). Antispasmodic drug. 64

dideoxycytidine (ddC) (Antivir). AIDS drug. 146

dideoxyinosine (ddI) (Antivir). AIDS drug. 146

diethylstilbestrol (Stilphostrol) (Chemo). Hormonal chemotherapy drug. 153

difenoxin (Motofen) (GI). Narcotic antidiarrheal drug. 64

Diflucan (Antifung). Oral antifungal/antiyeast drug. 54, 149

diflunisal (Dolobid) (Ortho). Nonsteroidal anti-inflammatory drug. 70, 136

Di-Gel (GI). Antacid. 61-62

Digibind (Cardio). Antidote for digitalis toxicity. 75, 86

Digitalis lanata (plant). 5, 74-75

digitalis toxicity. 75-76

digitoxin (Crystodigin) (Cardio). Digitalis-type drug for congestive heart failure. 75, 79

digoxin immune fab (Digibind) (Cardio). Antidote for digitalis toxicity. 75, 86

digoxin (Lanoxin, Lanoxicaps) (Cardio). Digitalis-type drug for congestive heart failure. 3, 20, 75

dihydroergotamine (D.H.E. 45) (Analges). Used for migraine headaches. 138

Dilantin (Neuro). Used for tonic-clonic seizures. 6, 20, 120-121

Dilaudid (Analges). Narcotic analgesic drug. 135

dilevalol (Unicard) (Cardio). Investigational nonselective beta blocker. 80

diltiazem (Cardizem) (Cardio). Calcium channel blocker used for angina and hypertension. 78, 82

diluent. 40

dimenhydrinate (Dramamine) (GI). Used for motion sickness. 66

Dimetane (ENT). Decongestant. 99

Dimetapp (ENT). Decongestant and antihistamine combination. 100

dinoprostone (Prostin E2) (Ob/Gyn). Prostaglandin used to abort fetus. 115

dinoprost (Prostin F2 Alpha) (Ob/Gyn). Prostaglandin used to abort fetus. 115

diphenhydramine (Benadryl) (ENT, GI). Antihistamine; used for motion sickness. 32, 66, 99

diphenhydramine (Benadryl) (Derm). Topical antihistamine. 54

diphenidol (Vontrol) (GI). Used for motion sickness. 66

diphenoxylate (Lomotil) (GI). Narcotic antidiarrheal drug. 64

dipivefrin (Propine) (Oph). Miotic drug for glaucoma. 105

Diprosone (Derm). Topical corticosteroid anti-inflammatory drug. 53

dipyridamole (Persantine) (Cardio, Hem). Used in thallium testing; anticoagulant. 86, 92

disinfectant. 40

disopyramide (Norpace) (Cardio). Antiarrhythmic drug. 79

Di-Spaz (GI). Antispasmodic drug. 64

distribution of drug. 29

disulfiram (Antabuse) (Psych). Used to deter alcohol consumption. 132

Diucardin (Uro). Thiazide diuretic. 57

Diupres (Cardio). Antihypertensive and diuretic. 84

Diurese (Uro). Thiazide diuretic. 57

diuretic
loop. 57
potassium-sparing (Uro). 57
potassium-wasting (Uro). 57
thiazide. 57

diuretics (Uro). Class of drugs which excrete excessive water and sodium; used as antihypertensive drugs. 57-58, 80

Diuril (Uro). Thiazide diuretic. 57

DM. Part of a trade name drug, indicating it contains dextromethorphan. 99

DNA, recombinant. 6, 17

dobutamine (Dobutrex) (Cardio). Vasopressor to treat hypotension. 90

Dobutrex (Cardio). Vasopressor to treat hypotension. 90

docusate (Colace, Surfak) (GI). Laxative. 65

Dolobid (Ortho). Nonsteroidal anti-inflammatory drug. 69, 136

Dolophine (Analges). Used to wean patients from narcotics. 135, 139

Domeboro (Derm). See *Burow's solution.* 55

domperidone (Motilium) (GI). Used for nausea after chemotherapy. 67

dopamine (neurotransmitter). 29, 36, 66, 121-122

dopamine (Intropin) (Cardio). Vasopressor to treat hypotension. 90

Donnatal (GI). Antispasmodic and sedative combination drug. 64

Doral (Sed/Hyp). Nonbarbiturate benzodiazepine drug for insomnia. 124

Doriden (Sed/Hyp). Nonbarbiturate drug for insomnia. 123

dosage calculations for elderly or pediatric patients. 47-48

dose
loading. 41
maintenance. 41
therapeutic. 20
toxic. 20

dothiepin (Prothiaden) (Psych). Investigational tricyclic antidepressant. 131

doxazosin mesylate (Cardura) (Cardio). An alpha₁ blocker for hypertension. 83

doxepin (Adapin, Sinequan) (Psych). Tricyclic antidepressant with antianxiety effect. 128, 131

Doxidan (GI). Laxative. 65

doxorubicin (Adriamycin, Rubrex) (Chemo). Antibiotic used only for chemotherapy. 67, 153

doxycycline (Vibramycin) (Antibio). Tetracycline-type antibiotic. 116-117, 144

Dracula. 4

dram. 6, 44

Dramamine (GI). Used for motion sickness. 66

Dristan (ENT). Decongestant and pain reliever combination. 100

Drixoral (ENT). Decongestant and antihistamine combination. 100

dronabinol (Marinol) (GI). Used for nausea after chemotherapy. 67

droperidol (Inapsine) (Anes). Preoperative or intraoperative sedative. 161

drops (drug measurement). 46

drug
definition of. 1
fat-soluble. 30-31
water-soluble. 30-31

drug design. 15-17

drug effects. 35-37

Drug Enforcement Administration (DEA). 10, 49-50.

drug forms. 21-23

drug holiday. 123

drug idiosyncrasy. 35

drug legislation. 8-11

drug names. Spelling of. 13-14
See also *chemical, generic, brand,* or *trade name.* 13-15

drug of choice. 40

drug sources. 15-17

drug tolerance. 40

DS (abbreviation for *double strength*); part of trade name of drug. 40

DTIC-Dome (Chemo). Chemotherapy drug. 67, 154

Dulcolax (GI). Laxative. 65

Duracap. Part of trade name of drug indicating it is a time-release capsule. 40

Duracillin (Antibio). Penicillin-type antibiotic. 141

Duramorph (Analges). Narcotic analgesic drug. 135

Duranest (Anes). Regional/spinal anesthetic drug. 159

Duraphyl (Resp). Bronchodilator. 95

Duraquin (Cardio). Antiarrhythmic drug. 79

Duration (ENT). Decongestant. 98

Duricef (Antibio). Cephalosporin antibiotic. 143

Duvoid (Uro). Urinary tract antispasmodic drug. 60

Dyazide (Uro). Potassium-wasting and potassium-sparing diuretic combination. 58

Dymelor (Endo). Oral antidiabetic drug. 110

DynaCirc (Cardio). Investigational calcium channel blocker drug. 82

Dynapen (Antibio). Penicillin-type antibiotic. 141

dyphylline (Lufyllin) (Resp). Bronchodilator. 94-95

Dyrenium (Uro). Potassium-sparing diuretic. 58

dysmenorrhea, drugs for (Ob/Gyn). 115

E, e

Easprin (Ortho). Nonsteroidal anti-inflammatory drug. 70, 136

echothiophate iodide (Oph). Miotic drug for glaucoma. 105

econazole (Spectazole) (Antifung). Topical antifungal/antiyeast drug. 54

Ecotrin (Ortho). Nonsteroidal anti-inflammatory drug. 21, 70, 136

Edecrin (Uro). Loop diuretic. 58

E.E.S. (Antibio). Erythromycin antibiotic. 117, 145

effect
allergic. 35
drug. 35-37
first-pass. 30
local drug. 32-33
negative chronotropic (Cardio). 74
positive inotropic (Cardio). 74
side. 32-34
systemic drug. 32-33
therapeutic drug. 18, 32-34
toxic drug. 18, 34

Ehrlich, Paul. 13

Elavil (Psych). Tricyclic antidepressant. 14, 131

Eldepryl (Neuro). Used to treat Parkinson disease. 122

elderly patients, drugs and. 30-31, 47-48

Eldisine (Chemo). Investigational chemotherapy drug. 153

elixir. 9, 22

Elixophyllin (Resp). Bronchodilator. 95

Elspar (Chemo). Chemotherapy drug. 154

Emcyt (Chemo). Hormonal chemotherapy drug. 153

emergency drugs for resuscitation. 27, 46, 88-91

Emete-Con (GI). Antiemetic. 66

Eminase (Cardio, Hem). Thrombolytic enzyme. 92

Empirin With Codeine (Analges). Narcotic analgesic drug. Empirin with 15 mg codeine, 30 mg codeine, or 60 mg codeine. 137

emulsion. 22

E-Mycin (Antibio). Erythromycin antibiotic. 117, 145

enalapril (Vasotec) (Cardio). ACE inhibitor drug used for hypertension. 82

encainide (Enkaid) (Cardio). Antiarrhythmic drug. 79

Endep (Psych). Tricyclic antidepressant. 131

endocrine drugs. 107-108

endometriosis, drugs for. 112

endorphin. 134

endotracheal administration of drugs. 88

Enduron (Uro). A thiazide diuretic. 57

Enduronyl (Cardio). Antihypertensive and diuretic combination. 84

enflurane (Ethrane) (Anes). Inhaled general anesthetic drug. 160

Enkaid (Cardio). Antiarrhythmic drug. 79

Enovid (Ob/Gyn). Used to treat hypermenorrhea. 118

enoxacin (Comprecin) (Antibio). Investigational antibiotic. 145

Entex LA (ENT). Decongestant and expectorant combination. 21, 100

Ephedra (plant). 4

ephedrine (ENT). Decongestant. 98

ephedrine (Resp). Bronchodilator. 4, 94

"epi" (a slang term for *epinephrine*).

Epifrin (Oph). Miotic drug for glaucoma. 105

epilepsy. 6, 20, 119, 120-121.

epinephrine (Adrenalin) (Cardio, Resp). Bronchodilator and cardiac stimulant. 46, 88-89, 94-95

epinephrine (Anes). Used with local anesthetic. 158

epinephrine (neurotransmitter). 36

epinephrine (Bronkaid Mist, Primatene Mist) (Resp). Over-the-counter bronchodilator. 94-95

epinephrine (Epifrin, Eppy/N) (Oph). Miotic drug for glaucoma. 105

Epitrate (Oph). Miotic drug for glaucoma. 105

epoetin alfa (Epogen) (Hem, Uro). Stimulates RBC production in patients with chronic renal failure. 60

Epogen (Hem, Uro). Stimulates RBC production in patients with chronic renal failure. 60

Eppy/N (Oph). Miotic drug for glaucoma. 105

Epsom salt (GI). Laxative. 65

Equagesic (Psych). Antianxiety drug and aspirin combination. 132, 139

Equanil (Psych). Antianxiety drug. 128

Ergamisol (Chemo). Chemotherapy drug. 155

ergonovine (Ergotrate) (Ob/Gyn). Used to slow postpartum bleeding. 112

ergotamine (Ergostat) (Analges). Used to treat migraine headaches. 138

Ergostat (Analges). Used to treat migraine headaches. 138

Ergotrate (Ob/Gyn). Used to slow postpartum bleeding. 112

ERYC (Antibio). Erythromycin antibiotic. 117, 145

Eryderm (Derm). Antiacne drug. 51

Erypar (Antibio). Erythromycin antibiotic. 145

EryPed (Antibio). Erythromycin antibiotic. 145

erythrityl tetranitrate (Cardilate) (Cardio). Antianginal drug. 77

erythromycin (Eryderm, Staticin) (Derm). Topical antiacne drug. 51, 53

erythromycin (E.E.S., ERYC, Ilosone) (Antibio). Oral antibiotic. 117, 145

erythromycin (Ilotycin) (Ophth) Topical antibiotic. 103, 117

Ery-Tab (Antibio). Erythromycin antibiotic. 145

Esidrix (Uro). Thiazide diuretic. 13-14, 57

Eskalith (Psych). Used for manic-depressive disorder. 132

esmolol (Brevibloc) (Cardio). Cardioselective beta blocker used for arrhythmia. 79

Estar (Derm). Coal tar gel for psoriasis. 52

estazolam (ProSom) (Sed/Hyp). Investigational nonbarbiturate drug for insomnia. 123

esterified estrogens (Estratab) (Ob/Gyn). Estrogen replacement for menopause. 114

Estinyl (Ob/Gyn). Estrogen replacement for menopause. 114

Estrace (Ob/Gyn). Estrogen replacement for menopause. 114

Estraderm (Ob/Gyn). Estrogen replacement for menopause. 114

estradiol cypionate (Depogen) (Ob/Gyn). Estrogen replacement for menopause. 114

estradiol (Estrace, Estraderm) (Ob/Gyn). Estrogen replacement for menopause. 114

Estradurin (Chemo). Hormonal chemotherapy drug. 153

estramustine (Emcyt) (Chemo). Hormonal chemotherapy drug. 153

Estratab (Ob/Gyn). Estrogen replacement for menopause. 114

estrogen. 113-114

estrogen replacement therapy. 114

estropipate (Ogen) (Ob/Gyn). Estrogen replacement for menopause. 114

Estrovis (Ob/Gyn) Estrogen replacement for menopause. 114

ethacrynic acid (Edecrin) (Uro). Loop diuretic. 58

ethambutol (Myambutol) (Resp). Antitubercular drug. 96

Ethamolin (GI). Sclerosing agent used to stop esophageal bleeding. 68

ethanolamine oleate (Ethamolin) (GI). Sclerosing agent used to stop esophageal bleeding. 68

ethchlorvynol (Placidyl) (Sed/Hyp). Nonbarbiturate drug for insomnia. 123

ether (Anes). 156-157

ethinamate (Valmid) (Sed/Hyp). Nonbarbiturate drug for insomnia. 123

ethinyl estradiol (Estinyl) (Ob/Gyn). Estrogen replacement for menopause. 114

Ethmozine (Cardio). Antiarrhythmic drug. 79

ethopropazine (Parsidol) (Neuro). Used to treat Parkinson disease. 123

ethosuximide (Zarontin) (Neuro). Used for absence seizures. 121

ethotoin (Peganone) (Neuro). Used for tonic-clonic seizures. 120-121

Ethrane (Anes). Inhaled general anesthetic. 160

etidocaine (Duranest) (Anes). Regional/ spinal anesthetic. 159

etodolac (Ultradol) (Ortho). Investigational nonsteroidal anti-inflammatory drug. 70, 138

etomidate (Amidate) (Anes). Intravenous agent for induction of general anesthesia. 159

etoposide (VP-16, VePesid) (Chemo). Chemotherapy drug. 153

Etrafon (Psych). Antipsychotic and anti-depressant combination. 132

etretinate (Tegison) (Derm). Oral drug for severe psoriasis. 52

Eulexin (Chemo). Hormonal chemotherapy drug. 153

Euthroid (Endo). Thyroid hormone replacement. 107

Evac-Q-Kit (GI) Bowel evacuant/bowel prep. 65

Excedrin (Analges). Nonaspirin analgesic, aspirin and caffeine combination drug. 137

excretion of drugs. 30-31

Exelderm (Derm). Topical antifungal drug. 54

Ex-Lax (GI). Laxative. 65

Exosurf (Resp). Investigational lung surfactant supplement for premature infants. 97

expectorants (ENT). Class of drugs which thin mucus to facilitate productive coughing. 40, 99

Extentab. Part of trade name of drug, indicating it is a time-release tablet. 40

■

F, f

5-aminosalicylic acid (GI). See *5-ASA*.

5-ASA (GI). Anti-inflammatory drug for ulcerative colitis. 65-66

5-FU (Chemo). Abbreviation for 5-fluorouracil. See *fluorouracil*.

famotidine (Pepcid) (GI). H$_2$ blocker to heal ulcers. 62

fat-soluble drug. 30-31

FDA (Food and Drug Administration).

Feen-a-Mint (GI). Laxative. 65

Feldene (Ortho). Nonsteroidal anti-inflammatory drug. 70, 138

Femstat (Ob/Gyn). Topical antiyeast drug for vaginal infections. 115

fenoprofen (Nalfon) (Ortho). Nonsteroidal anti-inflammatory drug. 70, 138

fenoterol HBr (Berotec) (Resp). Investigational bronchodilator. 94

fentanyl (Sublimaze) (Anes). Intravenous general anesthetic. 160

ferrous sulfate. 49

fetus, drug effects on. 29

FFP (fresh frozen plasma) (Hem). Given intravenously to replace plasma proteins and clotting factors. 164

Fiberall (GI). Laxative. 65

FiberCon (GI). Laxative. 65

Fiorinal (Analges). Analgesic containing aspirin and phenobarbital. 139

first-pass effect. 30

Flagyl (Antibio, Ob/Gyn). Antibiotic; oral amebicide drug for vaginal infections from Trichomonas. 116, 145

flavoxate (Urispas) (Uro). Antispasmodic. 59

Flaxedil (Anes). Intraoperative muscle-paralyzing drug. 160

flecainide (Tambocor) (Cardio). Antiarrhythmic drug. 79

Fleet enema (GI). 65

Fletcher's Castoria (GI). Laxative. 65

Flexeril (Ortho). Skeletal muscle relaxant. 72

Flexon (Ortho). Skeletal muscle relaxant. 72

Florinef (Endo). Used to treat Addison disease. 108

floxuridine (FUDR) (Chemo). Pyrimidine antagonist chemotherapy drug. 151

fluconazole (Diflucan) (Antifung). Oral antifungal/antiyeast drug. 54, 149

flucytosine (Ancobon) (Antifung). Oral antifungal/antiyeast drug. 149

fludrocortisone (Florinef) (Endo). Used to treat Addison disease. 108

Flumadine (Antivir). For influenza virus A. 148

flunisolide (AeroBid) (Resp). Inhaled corticosteroid. 95

flunisolide (Nasalide) (ENT). Intranasal corticosteroid. 101

fluocinolone (Lidex, Synalar) (Derm). Topical corticosteroid anti-inflammatory drug. 53

fluorescein (Oph). Yellow dye which shows corneal abrasions. 106

fluorouracil (5-FU, Adrucil) (Chemo). Pyrimidine antagonist chemotherapy drug. 151

Fluosol (Cardio). Oxygen-carrying solution for coronary artery surgery. 86

Fluothane (Anes). Inhaled general anesthetic drug. 158, 160

fluoxetine (Prozac) (Psych). Antidepressant. 131

fluphenazine (Prolixin) (Psych). Phenothiazine antipsychotic drug. 129

flupirtine (Analges). Non-narcotic analgesic, investigational. 139

flurandrenolide (Cordran) (Derm). Topical corticosteroid anti-inflammatory drug. 53

flurazepam (Dalmane) (Sed/Hyp). Non-barbiturate benzodiazepine drug for insomnia. 123

flurbiprofen (Ansaid, Ocufen) (Ortho, Oph). Oral and topical anti-inflammatory drug. 70, 106, 138

flutamide (Eulexin) (Chemo). Hormonal chemotherapy drug. 153

foam (drug form). 22

Folex (Chemo, Derm). Folic acid antagonist chemotherapy drug; for severe psoriasis. 52, 152

Follutein (Ob/Gyn). Ovulation-stimulating drug for infertility. 111

Food and Drug Administration (FDA). 9, 11, 13, 17, 19-21, 33

Food, Drug and Cosmetic Act. 9

Forane (Anes). Inhaled general anesthetic. 160

forms, drug. 21-23

Formula 44 (ENT). Decongestant and non-narcotic antitussive combination. 100

Fortaz (Antibio). Third-generation cephalosporin antibiotic. 143

foscarnet (Antivir). AIDS drug. 146

Fostex (Derm). Topical over-the-counter acne preparation. 51

foxglove (plant). 3, 74-75

fresh frozen plasma (FFP) (Hem). Given intravenously to replace plasma proteins and clotting factors. 164

Frisium (Psych). Investigational benzodiazepine drug for anxiety. 127

FUDR (Chemo). Abbreviation for floxuridine. 151

Fulvicin (Antifung). Oral antifungal drug. 149

Fungizone (Antifung). Oral antifungal/anti-yeast drug. 149

Furacin (Derm). Topical antibiotic for burns. 56

Furadantin (Uro). Urinary tract antibiotic. 59

furosemide (Lasix) (Uro). Loop diuretic. 58

■

G, g

g (gram). 44-45

gallamine triethiodide (Flaxedil) (Anes). Intraoperative muscle-paralyzing drug. 160

gallstones, drugs for. 68

ganciclovir (Cytovene) (Antivir). Used for cytomegalovirus. 148

Gantanol (Antibio). Sulfonamide anti-infective drug. 59, 140, 144

Gantrisin (Antibio). Sulfonamide anti-infective drug. 59, 140

Garamycin (Antibio). Aminoglycoside antibiotic. 26, 30, 34, 144

Garamycin (Derm, Oph). Topical and ophthalmic antibiotic. 53, 103, 117

Gardnerella vaginalis. 115

Gastrocrom (GI). Oral mast cell inhibitor for food allergies. 68

Gastrozepine (GI). Investigational antiulcer drug. 63

Gas-X (GI). Antiflatulent drug. 62

gauge of needle. 41

Gelusil (GI). Antacid. 61-62

gemfibrozil (Lopid) (Cardio). Used to treat hypertriglyceridemia. 85

Gemonil (Neuro). Barbiturate for tonic-clonic and absence seizures. 120-121

gene splicing. 17

generic drug names. 13, 19-20, 49

genetic engineering. 17

Genoptic (Oph). Topical antibiotic for eye. 103

gentamicin (Garamycin, Genoptic) (Oph). Topical antibiotic for eye. 103

gentamicin (Garamycin) (Antibio, Derm). Topical and oral aminoglycoside antibiotic. 34, 53, 144

gentian violet (Derm). Topical antibacterial and antifungal dye. 55

Gentran 40, Gentran 75 (Hem). Plasma volume expander. 165

Geopen (Antibio). Penicillin-type antibiotic. 116, 141

glaucoma. 25, 104

glipizide (Glucotrol) (Endo). Oral antidiabetic drug. 110

Glucotrol (Endo). Oral antidiabetic drug. 110

glutamic acid (Acidulin) (GI). Gastric acid replacement. 68

glutethimide (Doriden) (Sed/Hyp). Non-barbiturate drug for insomnia. 123

glyburide (DiaBeta, Micronase) (Endo). Oral antidiabetic drug. 110

glycerin. 23

glycopyrrolate (Robinul) (GI). Antispasmodic drug. 64

gold salts (Ortho). Used for arthritis. 71

gold sodium thiomalate (Myochrysine) (Ortho). Gold salts used for arthritis. 71

GoLytely (or GoLYTELY) (GI). Bowel evacuant used prior to surgery. 65

gonadorelin (Lutrepulse) (Ob/Gyn). Used to treat amenorrhea. 114

goserelin (Zoladex) (Chemo). Hormonal chemotherapy drug. 153

gout, drugs for. 72

gr. (grain). 6, 44

grain (gr.). 6, 44

gram (g). 44-45

gram-negative bacteria. 144

gram-positive bacteria. 144

Grifulvin (Antifung). Oral antifungal drug. 54, 149

Grisactin (Antifung). Oral antifungal drug. 149

griseofulvin (Fulvicin, Grifulvin, Grisactin) (Antifung). Oral antifungal drug. 54, 149

gt (drop), gtt (drops). 46

guaifenesin (Robitussin, Naldecon) (ENT). Expectorant. 99

guanabenz (Wytensin) (Cardio). Antihypertensive drug. 83

guanadrel (Hylorel) (Cardio). Antihypertensive drug. 83

guanethidine (Ismelin) (Cardio). Antihypertensive drug. 83

guanfacine (Tenex) (Cardio). Antihypertensive drug. 83

gutta, guttae. See *gt.*

Gyne-Lotrimin (Ob/Gyn). Topical antiyeast drug for vaginal infections. 115

Gyrocaps. Part of the trade name of a drug; it indicates a slow-release capsule. 40

■

H, h

H₁ **receptor.** 36, 63, 99

H₂ **blockers** (GI). Class of drugs which block histamine release in the stomach to decrease acid production. 62

H₂ **receptor.** 36, 62-63

Haemophilus vaginalis. 115

halazepam (Paxipam) (Psych). Benzodiazepine antianxiety drug. 13, 127

halcinonide (Halog) (Derm). Topical corticosteroid anti-inflammatory drug. 53

Halcion (Sed/Hyp). Nonbarbiturate benzodiazepine drug for insomnia. 124

Haldol (Psych). Antipsychotic drug. 6, 14, 129

Haldrone (Endo). Steroidal anti-inflammatory drug. 108

half-life. 9, 40, 75

half normal saline. Intravenous fluid of 0.45% NaCl. 163

Halog (Derm). Topical corticosteroid anti-inflammatory drug. 53

haloperidol (Haldol) (Psych). Antipsychotic drug. 14, 129

haloprogin (Halotex) (Derm). Topical antifungal drug. 54

Halotex (Derm). Topical antifungal drug. 54

halothane (Fluothane) (Anes). Inhaled general anesthetic. 35, 158, 160

Haltran (Ob/Gyn). Over-the-counter drug for dysmenorrhea. 115

Hamlet. 4

Harmonyl (Cardio). Antihypertensive drug. 83

Harrison Narcotics Act. 10

HCG or hCG (Ob/Gyn). Abbreviation for human chorionic gonadotropin. 111

HCTZ (Uro). Abbreviation for hydrochlorothiazide. 57

Healon (Oph). Aqueous humor replacement. 106

Hemabate (Ob/Gyn). Prostaglandin used to abort fetus. 115

henbane (plant). 4

heparin (Calciparine) (Hem). Anticoagulant. 26, 92

heparin lock. 162

heroin. 8, 10, 135, 139

herpes simplex virus. 146, 148

Herplex Liquifilm (Oph). Topical antiviral drug for eye. 104

Hespan (Hem). Plasma volume expander. 165

hetastarch (Hespan) (Hem). Plasma volume expander. 165

Hibiclens (Derm). Topical antibacterial scrub. 56

Hiprex (Uro). Used for urinary tract infections. 59

Hismanal (ENT). Decongestant. 99

histamine. 35, 62, 99

homatropine (Oph). Mydriatic drug. 105

hormone, chemotherapy (Chemo). Class of chemotherapy drugs. 153

household measurement of drugs. 46

h.s. (hour of sleep, at bedtime).

human chorionic gonadotropin (HCG or hCG, Follutein) (Ob/Gyn). Stimulates ovulation to treat infertility. 111

Humatrope (Endo). Growth hormone replacement. 107

Humorsol (Oph). Miotic drug for glaucoma. 105

Humulin 70/30 (Endo). 70% NPH plus 30% regular insulin. 110

Humulin BR (Endo). Injectable regular insulin. 109

Humulin L (Endo). Injectable lente insulin. 109

Humulin N (Endo). Injectable NPH insulin. 109

Humulin R (Endo). Injectable regular insulin. 109

Humulin U (Endo). Injectable ultralente insulin. 109

hyaluronidase (Wydase). Given in conjunction with other drugs to improve their absorption.

Hycodan (ENT). Narcotic antitussive drug. 99, 134

Hycomine (ENT). Decongestant, antihistamine, narcotic antitussive, pain reliever combination drug. 100

Hycort (Derm). Topical corticosteroid anti-inflammatory drug. 53

hydantoins (Neuro). Class of drugs used to treat epilepsy. 120

Hydergine (Psych). Used for Alzheimer disease. 133

hydralazine (Apresoline) (Cardio). Vasodilator. 83

hydroxyzine (Vistaril) (Anes). Preoperative drug to sedate and relieve anxiety.

Hydergine (Psych). Used for Alzheimer disease.

hydralazine (Apresoline) (Cardio). Vasodilator. 83

Hydrea (Chemo). Chemotherapy drug. 154

hydrochlorothiazide (Esidrix, HydroDIURIL, Oretic) (Uro). Thiazide diuretic. 13, 57

hydrocodone (Hycodan) (ENT). Narcotic antitussive. 99

hydrocortisone (Cortaid, Hycort) (Derm). Topical corticosteroid anti-inflammatory drug. 52-53

hydrocortisone (Cortef, Solu-Cortef) (Endo, Ortho). Oral corticosteroid anti-inflammatory drug. 71, 108

hydrocortisone (Cortenema, Cortifoam) (GI). Topical corticosteroid anti-inflammatory drug for ulcerative colitis. 66

Hydrocortone (Endo, Ortho). Oral corticosteroid anti-inflammatory drug. 71, 108

hydrocyanic acid. 8

HydroDIURIL (Uro). Thiazide diuretic. 13, 57

hydroflumethiazide (Saluron) (Uro). Thiazide diuretic. 57

hydromorphone (Dilaudid) (Analges). Narcotic analgesic. 135

Hydromox (Uro). Thiazide diuretic. 57

Hydromox R (Cardio). Antihypertensive and diuretic. 84

hydroxyprogesterone (Hylutin) (Ob/Gyn). Used to treat amenorrhea. 114

hydroxyurea (Hydrea) (Chemo). Chemotherapy drug. 154

hydroxyzine (Vistaril) (Anes). Preoperative drug to sedate and relieve anxiety. 161

Hygroton (Uro). Diuretic. 57

Hylorel (Cardio). Antihypertensive drug. 83

Hylutin (Ob/Gyn). Used to treat amenorrhea. 114

hyperactivity, drugs for. 124

hypercholesterolemia, drugs for. 85

hyperlipidemia. 84

Hyperstat (Cardio). Used for hypertensive crisis.

hypertriglyceridemia, drugs for. 85-86

Hyperstat (Cardio). Used for hypertensive crisis. 82

hypertension. 6, 10, 19, 80-82.

hypertensive crisis. 82

hyperthermia, malignant. 35

hypnotic drugs. 123-124

hypodermic. 40

Hyskon (Ob/Gyn). Fluid used intraoperatively to facilitate visualization of uterus. 118

Hytone (Derm). Topical corticosteroid anti-inflammatory drug. 53

Hytrin (Cardio). An alpha$_1$ blocker antihypertensive drug. 83

■

I, i

ibuprofen (Advil, Medipren, Nuprin) (Analges, Ob/Gyn, Ortho). Over-the-counter nonsteroidal anti-inflammatory drug. 70, 138

ibuprofen (Motrin, Rufen) (Analges, Ob/Gyn, Ortho). Used to treat dysmenorrhea; nonsteroidal anti-inflammatory drug. 70, 115, 138

idiosyncrasy, drug. 35

idoxuridine (Herplex Liquifilm) (Oph). Topical antiviral drug. 104

Ifex (Chemo). Alkylating chemotherapy drug. 152

ifosfamide (Ifex) (Chemo). Alkylating chemotherapy drug. 152

Ilopan (GI). Gastric stimulant. 66

Ilosone (Antibio). Erythromycin antibiotic. 145

Ilotycin (Antibio). Erythromycin antibiotic. 117, 145

Ilotycin (Oph). Topical antibiotic for eye. 103, 117

I.M. (intramuscular). 26

imipramine (Tofranil) (Psych). Tricyclic antidepressant. 131

Imodium (GI). Narcotic antidiarrheal drug. 64

Inapsine (Anes). Preoperative or intraoperative sedative. 161

inch (drug measurement). 45

indecainide (Decabid) (Cardio). Antiarrhythmic drug. 79

Inderal (Cardio, Analges). Nonselective beta blocking drug used for angina, hypertension, arrhythmia; used to prevent migraine headaches. 6, 10, 19, 77, 79-80, 139

Inderide (Cardio). Antihypertensive and diuretic combination. 84

index, therapeutic. 18, 20, 34, 43

Indocin (Cardio, Ortho). Given intravenously to close patent ductus arteriosus in newborn infants; nonsteroidal anti-inflammatory drug. 19, 70, 72, 86

induction of anesthesia. 159

indomethacin (Indocin) (Cardio, Ortho). Given intravenously to close patent ductus arteriosus in newborn infants; nonsteroidal anti-inflammatory drug. 19, 70, 72, 86

inert ingredients in drugs. 20

infants. See pediatric patients.

Infatab. Part of trade name of drug, indicating it is a chewable tablet in pediatric dose. 41

infertility, drugs for. 111

Inflamase (Oph). Topical corticosteroid. 104

INH (Resp). Abbreviation for chemical name of isoniazid. 96

inhalation, administration by. 25, 28

inhaler, metered-dose (Pulm). Device for inhaling drugs into lungs. 94

Innovar (Anes). Fentanyl and droperidol combination drug. 161

Inocor (Cardio). Non-digitalis drug used for congestive heart failure. 75

inotropic effect, positive. 74

insomnia, drugs for. 123-124

Insulatard NPH (Endo). Injectable NPH insulin. 109

insulin. 6, 26, 45, 109-110

insulin, human. 6, 17

insulin syringe. 41

Intal (Resp). Mast cell inhibitor for bronchial asthma. 95-96

interaction
  drug-drug. 37
  drug-food. 37

interferon alfa-2a (Roferon-A) (Antivir, Chemo). AIDS drug; chemotherapy drug. 146

interferon alfa-2b (Intron A) (Antivir, Chemo, Derm, Gyn). AIDS and chemotherapy drug. Injected for herpes genital lesions. 54, 117, 146

interferon alfa-n3 (Alferon N) (Chemo, Derm, Gyn). Chemotherapy drug; also injected drug for herpes genital lesions. 54, 117

interferon beta (Betaseron) (Antivir). AIDS drug. 146
international unit (IU). 45
intra-arterial administration. 26
intra-articular administration. 26
intracardiac administration. 26, 46, 89
intradermal administration. 25
intramuscular administration. 26
Intralipid. Intravenous fat solution. 22, 163
intrathecal administration. 26
intravenous (I.V.) administration. 26, 88. See also *I.V.*
intravenous fluids/solutions. 162-163
intravenous lipids (Intralipid, Liposyn). Intravenous fat solution. 163
Intron A (Antivir, Chemo, Derm, Gyn). AIDS and chemotherapy drug. Also injected drug for herpes genital lesions. 54, 117, 146, 155
Intropin (Cardio). Vasopressor to treat hypotension. 90
in vitro drug testing. 17
in vivo drug testing. 17
Iopidine (Oph). Miotic drug for glaucoma. 105
ipratropium (Atrovent) (Resp). Bronchodilator. 94
Ismelin (Cardio). Antihypertensive drug. 83
isocarboxazid (Marplan) (Psych). MAO inhibitor antidepressant drug. 131
isoetharine (Bronkometer, Bronkosol) (Resp). Bronchodilator. 94
isoflurane (Forane) (Anes). Inhaled general anesthetic. 160

isomer. 41
isoniazid (INH, Nydrazid) (Resp). Antitubercular drug. 96
isoprinosine (Antivir). AIDS drug. 146
isoproterenol (Isuprel, Medihaler-Iso) (Cardio, Resp). Vasopressor for hypotension; bronchodilator. 90, 94
Isoptin (Cardio, Analges). Calcium channel blocker drug for angina, arrhythmias, and hypertension; also for migraine headaches. 78-79, 139
Isordil (Cardio). Antianginal drug. 77
isosorbide dinitrate (Isordil) (Cardio). Antianginal drug. 77
isotretinoin (Accutane) (Derm). Oral drug for acne. 52
isoxicam (Maxicam) (Ortho). Investigational nonsteroidal anti-inflammatory drug. 70, 138
isoxsuprine (Vasodilan) (Cardio). Peripheral vasodilating drug. 84
isradipine (DynaCirc) (Cardio). Investigational calcium channel blocker drug. 82
Isuprel (Cardio, Resp). Vasopressor for hypotension; bronchodilator. 90, 94
IU (international unit). 45
I.V. (intravenous) administration. 26, 88
I.V. drip. 26, 88, 162
I.V. piggyback. 26, 162
I.V. port. 26, 162
I.V. push. 26, 88, 162

■

K, k

Kabikinase (Cardio, Hem). Thrombolytic enzyme. 92

kanamycin (Kantrex) (Antibio). Aminoglycoside antibiotic. 28, 34, 144

Kantrex (Antibio). Aminoglycoside antibiotic. 34, 144

Kaolin (GI). Antidiarrheal drug. 64

Kaopectate (GI). Antidiarrheal drug. 64

Kapseal. Part of the trade name of drug, indicating it is a time-release capsule. 40

Kay Ciel (Uro). Potassium supplement taken with diuretics. 58

K-Dur (Uro). Potassium supplement taken with diuretics. 58

K-Lor (Uro). Potassium supplement taken with diuretics. 58

Keflex (Antibio). First-generation cephalosporin antibiotic. 35, 143

Keflin (Antibio). First-generation cephalosporin antibiotic. 143

Keftab (Antibio). First-generation cephalosporin antibiotic. 143

Kefurox (Antibio). Second-generation cephalosporin antibiotic. 143

Kefzol (Antibio). First-generation cephalosporin antibiotic. 143

Kemadrin (Neuro). Used to treat Parkinson disease. 123

Kenacort (Endo, Ortho). Oral corticosteroid anti-inflammatory drug. 71, 108

Kenalog (Derm). Topical corticosteroid anti-inflammatory drug. 22, 46, 53

Kenalog (Endo). Oral corticosteroid anti-inflammatory drug. 108

Kenalog in Orabase (ENT). Topical corticosteroid anti-inflammatory drug for mouth. 101

Keri (Derm). Topical lotion. 22

Kerlone (Cardio). Cardioselective beta blocker drug used for hypertension. 81

Ketalar (Anes). Intravenous drug for induction of general anesthesia. 159

ketamine (Ketalar) (Anes). Intravenous drug for induction of general anesthesia. 159

ketoconazole (Nizoral) (Antifung). Topical and oral antifungal/antiyeast drug. 54, 149

ketoprofen (Orudis) (Ob/Gyn, Ortho). Used to treat dysmenorrhea; nonsteroidal anti-inflammatory drug. 70, 115, 138

ketorolac (Toradol) (Analges). Nonsteroidal anti-inflammatory drug. 70, 138

ketotifen (Zaditen) (Resp). Investigational mast cell inhibitor. 96

kg (kilogram). 44-45

kidney. 30, 57

kilogram (kg). 44-45

Klonopin (Neuro). Used to treat absence seizures. 121

Klorvess (Uro). Potassium supplement taken with diuretics. 21, 58

Klotrix (Uro). Potassium supplement taken with diuretics. 58

K-Lyte (Uro). Potassium supplement taken with diuretics. 58

K-Tab (Uro). Potassium supplement taken with diuretics. 58

Kwell (Derm). Topical drug for scabies or mites. 55

■

L, l

L-asparaginase (Chemo). Chemotherapy drug. 155

L-dopa (Neuro). Used to treat Parkinson disease. 122

L-hyoscyamine (Anaspaz, Levsin) (GI). Used for GI spasm. 59, 64

LA (abbreviation for *long-acting*). Part of the trade name of a drug. 21, 41

labetalol (Normodyne, Trandate) (Cardio). Alpha and beta blocker used for hypertension. 80

lactulose (GI). Laxative. 65

Lacrisert (Oph). Artificial tears. 106

lactated Ringer's (LR). Intravenous fluid of dextrose, electrolytes, and normal saline. 163

lanolin. 5, 22

Lanoxicaps (Cardio). Digitalis drug for congestive heart failure. 75

Lanoxin (Cardio). Digitalis drug for congestive heart failure. 3, 20, 75

Larodopa (Neuro). Used to treat Parkinson disease. 122

Larotid (Antibio). Penicillin-type antibiotic. 116, 141

Lasix (Uro). Loop diuretic. 58

law, drug. See *legislation, drug.*

laxative
 bulk-producing. 65
 irritant. 65
 magnesium. 65
 mechanical. 65
 softener. 65

laxatives (GI). Class of drugs used to relieve constipation. 64-65

legislation, drug. 8-11

Lente Iletin (Endo). Injectable lente insulin. 109

lente insulin (Lente Iletin, Humulin L) (Endo). Injectable lente insulin. 109

Leukeran (Chemo). Alkylating chemotherapy drug. 152

leuprolide (Lupron) (Chemo). Hormonal chemotherapy drug. 153

levamisole (Ergamisol) (Chemo). Chemotherapy drug. 155

Levatol (Cardio). Nonselective beta blocker drug used for hypertension. 80

level
 peak drug. 42
 trough drug. 42

levobunolol (Betagan) (Oph). Beta blocker drug for glaucoma. 105

levodopa (L-dopa, Larodopa) (Neuro). Used to treat Parkinson disease. 6, 29, 122

Levo-Dromoran (Analges). Narcotic analgesic drug. 135

Levophed (Cardio). Vasopressor for hypotension. 90

levorotary. 41

levorphanol (Levo-Dromoran) (Analges). Narcotic analgesic drug. 135

levothyroxine (Synthroid) (Endo). Thyroid hormone replacement. 107

Levsin (GI). Antispasmodic drug. 64

Librax (Psych, GI). Antianxiety and GI antispasmodic combination. 64, 132

Librium (Psych, Neuro). Benzodiazepine-type antianxiety drug; also for alcohol withdrawal seizures. 6, 10, 15, 125, 127

lice. 55

Lidex (Derm). Topical corticosteroid anti-inflammatory drug. 53

lidocaine (Xylocaine) (Derm, ENT). Topical anesthetic. 32, 102, 158

lidocaine (Xylocaine) (Anes). Local/regional/spinal anesthetic. 32, 158

lidocaine (Xylocaine) (Cardio). Antiarrhythmic drug. 24, 30, 32, 79-80, 88, 90, 157, 159

Limbitrol DS (Psych). Antianxiety and antidepressant combination. 132

Lincocin (Antibio). Antibiotic. 145

lincomycin (Lincocin) (Antibio). Antibiotic. 145

lindane (Kwell) (Derm). Topical drug for scabies or mites. 55

Lioresal (Ortho). For severe muscle spasticity. 72

liothyronine (Cytomel) (Endo). Thyroid hormone replacement. 107

liotrix (Euthroid, Thyrolar) (Endo). Thyroid hormone replacement. 107

Liposyn. Intravenous fat solution. 163

Liquifilm (Oph). Artificial tears. 106

Liquiprin (Analges). Nonaspirin analgesic drug. 137

lisinopril (Prinivil, Zestril) (Cardio). ACE inhibitor drug used for hypertension. 82

lithium (Eskalith, Lithobid, Lithotabs) (Antivir, Psych). AIDS drug; also for manic-depressive disorder. 132, 147

Lithobid (Psych, Antivir). For manic-depressive disorder; an AIDS drug. 132, 147

Lithotabs (Psych, Antivir). For manic-depressive disorder; an AIDS drug. 132, 147

liver. 30

loading dose. 41

local drug effect. 32-33

Lodosyn (Neuro). Used to treat Parkinson disease. 122

Loestrin 1.5/30 (Ob/Gyn) Combination progesterone/estrogen oral contraceptive. 113

Loestrin 1/20 (Ob/Gyn) Combination progesterone/estrogen oral contraceptive. 113

Lomotil (GI). Narcotic antidiarrheal drug. 10, 64

lomustine (CeeNu) (Chemo). Alkylating chemotherapy drug.

Loniten (Cardio). Vasodilator. 83

loop diuretic (Uro). Diuretic acting at the loop of Henle. 57-58

Lo/Ovral (Ob/Gyn). Combination progesterone/estrogen oral contraceptive. 113

loperamide (Imodium) (GI). Narcotic antidiarrheal drug. 64

Lopid (Cardio). For hypertriglyceridemia. 85

Lopressor (Cardio, Analges). Cardioselective beta blocker drug used for hypertension and angina; also used for migraine headaches. 77, 79, 81, 138

Loprox (Derm). Topical antifungal agent. 54

loratadine (Claritin) (ENT). Investigational decongestant. 99

lorazepam (Ativan) (Psych). Benzodiazepine-type antianxiety drug. 13, 127

Lorelco (Cardio). Used for hypercholesterolemia. 85

Losec (GI). Decreases gastric acid. 68

lotion. 22

Lotrimin (Derm). Topical antifungal agent. 54

Lotusate (Neuro). Barbiturate hypnotic drug for sleep. 124

lovastatin (Mevacor) (Cardio). Used for hypercholesterolemia. 85

loxapine (Loxitane) (Psych). Antipsychotic drug. 129

Loxitane (Psych). Antipsychotic drug. 129

lozenge. 21

LR (lactated Ringer's). Intravenous fluid of dextrose, electrolytes, and normal saline. 163

Ludiomil (Psych). Tetracyclic antidepressant. 130-131

Lufyllin (Resp). Bronchodilator. 94-95

Luminal (Neuro). Used for tonic-clonic seizures. 120-121

Lupron (Chemo). Hormonal chemotherapy drug. 153

Lutrepulse (Ob/Gyn). Used to treat amenorrhea. 114

lypressin (Diapid) (Endo). Used to treat diabetes insipidus. 108

M, m

Maalox (GI). Antacid. 22, 61

Maalox Plus (GI). Antacid and antigas combination drug.

Maalox II (GI). Antacid and anti-gas combination drug. 62

Macrodantin (Uro). Urinary tract antibiotic. 59

Macrodex (Hem). Plasma volume expander. 165

mafenide (Sulfamylon) (Derm). Topical antibacterial for burns. 56

"magic bullet." 13

magnesium sulfate (Ob/Gyn) Used for seizures in preeclampsia. 118

maintenance dose. 41

major tranquilizer (Psych). Class of drugs used for psychosis. 128-129

Mandelamine (Uro). Used for urinary tract infections. 59

Mandol (Antibio). Second-generation cephalosporin antibiotic. 143

mannitol (Osmitrol) (Neuro, Uro). Diuretic for renal failure and to decrease cerebral edema. 58, 125

MAO inhibitors (Psych). Class of drugs which inhibit monoamine oxidase enzyme; antidepressants. 37, 130-131

maprotiline (Ludiomil) (Psych). Tetracyclic antidepressant. 130-131

Marax (Resp). Bronchodilator and sedative combination. 95

Marcaine (Anes). Local/regional/spinal anesthetic. 158-159

Marcaine (Oph, Ortho). Local anesthetic for the eye or joints. 72, 106

Marinol (GI). Used for nausea after chemotherapy. 67

Marplan (Psych). MAO inhibitor antidepressant. 131

Mast cell inhibitor (Resp). Inhibits mast cells' role in allergic symptoms. 95-96

Matulane (Chemo). Chemotherapy drug. 155

Maxair (Resp). Bronchodilator. 94

Maxicam (Ortho). Investigational nonsteroidal anti-inflammatory drug. 70, 138

Maxidex (Oph). Topical corticosteroid for the eye. 104

Maxitrol (Oph). Topical corticosteroid/antibiotic combination. 104

Maxzide (Uro). Potassium-wasting and potassium-sparing combination diuretic. 58

May apple (plant). 153

mcg (microgram). 44-45

meadow saffron (plant). 4

Mebaral (Neuro). Barbiturate for tonic-clonic and absence seizures. 120-121

mechlorethamine (nitrogen mustard, Mustargen) (Chemo). Alkylating chemotherapy drug. 152

Meclan (Derm). Topical antibiotic for acne. 51

meclizine (Antivert, Bonine) (ENT). Used for motion sickness, vertigo. 67

meclocycline (Meclan) (Derm). Topical antibiotic for acne. 51

meclofenamate (Meclomen) (Ortho). Nonsteroidal anti-inflammatory drug. 70, 138

Meclomen (Ortho). Nonsteroidal anti-inflammatory drug. 70, 138

medicine, definition of. 1

Medihaler-Iso (Resp). Bronchodilator. 94

Medipren (Analges, Ob/Gyn, Ortho). Nonsteroidal anti-inflammatory drug. 70, 138

Medrol (Endo, Ortho). Oral corticosteroid anti-inflammatory drug. 71, 108

Medrol Enpak (GI). For ulcerative colitis. 66

medroxyprogesterone (Depo-Provera) (Chemo). Hormonal chemotherapy drug. 153

medroxyprogesterone (Provera) (Ob/Gyn). Used to treat amenorrhea. 114

mefenamic acid (Ponstel) (Ob/Gyn). Used to treat dysmenorrhea. 115

Mefoxin (Antibio). Second-generation cephalosporin antibiotic. 116, 143

Megace (Chemo). Hormonal chemotherapy drug. 153

megestrol (Megace) (Chemo). Hormonal chemotherapy drug. 153

Mellaril (Psych). Phenothiazine antipsychotic drug. 129

melphalan (Alkeran) (Chemo). Alkylating chemotherapy drug. 152

Menest (Ob/Gyn) Estrogen replacement for menopause. 114

menotropins (Pergonal) (Ob/Gyn). Ovulation-stimulating drug for infertility. 111

Menrium (Ob/Gyn). Estrogen and antianxiety combination drug for menopause. 114

meperidine (Demerol) (Anes). Preoperative drug to sedate, relieve pain. 135, 161

mephentermine (Wyamine) (Anes). Used to treat hypotension from spinal anesthesia. 161

mephenytoin (Mesantoin) (Neuro). Used for tonic-clonic seizures. 120-121

mephobarbital (Mebaral) (Neuro). Barbiturate for tonic-clonic and absence seizures. 120-121

Mephyton (Hem). Reverses oral anticoagulant overdose; also prophylactic against bleeding. 93

mepivacaine (Carbocaine) (Anes). Local/regional anesthetic. 158-159

meprobamate (Equanil, Miltown) (Psych). Antianxiety drug. 6, 128

Meprospan (Psych). Antianxiety drug. 128

mEq (milliequivalent). 46

mercaptopurine (Purinethol) (Chemo). Purine antagonist chemotherapy drug. 151

Merthiolate (Derm). Topical antiseptic. 22

mesalamine (Rowasa) (GI). Topical anti-inflammatory for ulcerative colitis. 65

Mesantoin (Neuro). Used for tonic-clonic seizures. 120-121

mesoridazine (Serentil) (Psych). Phenothiazine antipsychotic drug. 129

metabolism of drug. 29

metabolite. 29-30

Metamucil (GI). Laxative. 22, 28, 65

Metaprel (Resp). Bronchodilator. 94-95

metaproterenol (Alupent, Metaprel) (Resp). Bronchodilator. 94-95

metaraminol (Aramine) (Anes). Used for hypotension from spinal anesthesia. 161

metaxalone (Skelaxin) (Ortho). Skeletal muscle relaxant. 72

methacycline (Rondomycin) (Antibio). Tetracycline-type antibiotic. 116-117, 144

methadone (Dolophine) (Analges). Used to wean patients from narcotics. 135, 139

methamphetamine (Desoxyn) (Neuro). For attention deficit disorder, a CNS stimulant. 124

metharbital (Gemonil) (Neuro). Barbiturate for tonic-clonic, absence seizure. 120-121

methenamine (Hiprex, Mandelamine) (Uro). Used for urinary tract infections. 59

Methergine (Ob/Gyn) Used to slow postpartum bleeding. 112

methicillin (Staphcillin) (Antibio). Penicillin-type antibiotic. 141

methimazole (Tapazole) (Endo). Used to treat hyperthyroidism. 107

methocarbamol (Robaxin) (Ortho). Skeletal muscle relaxant. 72

methohexital (Brevital) (Anes). Intravenous barbiturate for induction of general anesthesia. 159

methotrexate (Folex) (Derm). Used for severe psoriasis. 52

methotrexate (Folex) (Chemo). Folic acid antagonist chemotherapy drug. 152

methotrexate (Rheumatrex) (Ortho). Used for severe arthritis. 71

methoxamine (Vasoxyl) (Anes). Used for hypotension from spinal anesthesia. 161

methoxsalen (Oxsoralen) (Derm). For severe, disabling psoriasis. 52

methoxyflurane (Penthrane) (Anes). Inhaled general anesthetic. 160

methscopolamine (Pamine) (GI). Antispasmodic drug. 64

methsuximide (Celontin) (Neuro). Used for absence seizures. 121

methyclothiazide (Enduron) (Uro). Thiazide diuretic. 57

methylergonovine (Methergine) (Ob/Gyn). Used to slow postpartum bleeding. 112

methyldopa (Aldomet) (Cardio). Antihypertensive agent. 83

methylphenidate (Ritalin) (Neuro). Used for attention deficit disorder, a CNS stimulant. 124

methylprednisolone (Depo-Medrol) (Endo, Ortho). Oral corticosteroid anti-inflammatory drug. 71, 108

methylprednisolone (Medrol Enpak) (GI). Topical corticosteroid anti-inflammatory drug for ulcerative colitis. 66

methyprylon (Noludar) (Sed/Hyp). Non-barbiturate drug for short-term insomnia. 124

methysergide (Sansert) (Analges). Used for migraine headaches. 138

metoclopramide (Reglan) (GI). Gastric stimulant. 66-67

metocurine (Metubine) (Anes). Intraoperative muscle-paralyzing drug. 160

metolazone (Zaroxolyn) (Uro). Diuretic. 57

metoprolol (Lopressor) (Cardio, Analges). Cardioselective beta blocker drug used for hypertension and angina; also used for migraine headaches. 77, 79, 81, 138

metric system. 44-46

Metrodin (Ob/Gyn). Ovulation-stimulating drug for infertility. 111

MetroGel (Derm). Topical drug for acne rosacea. 52

metronidazole (Flagyl) (Antibio, Ob/Gyn). Antibiotic and amebicide for *Trichomonas* vaginal infection. 116, 145

metronidazole (MetroGel) (Derm). Topical drug for acne rosacea. 52

Metubine (Anes). Intraoperative muscle-paralyzing drug. 160

Mevacor (Cardio). Used for hypercholesterolemia. 85

mexiletine (Mexitil) (Cardio). Antiarrhythmic drug. 79

Mexitil (Cardio). Antiarrhythmic drug. 79

Mezlin (Antibio). Penicillin-type antibiotic. 116, 141

mezlocillin (Mezlin) (Antibio). Penicillin-type antibiotic. 116, 141

mg (milligram). 44-45

mg/kg/day (milligrams of drug per kilograms of body weight per day).

mg/m² (milligrams of drug per square meter of body surface area).

Micatin (Derm). Topical antifungal drug. 54

miconazole (Micatin) (Derm). Topical antifungal drug. 54

miconazole (Monistat i.v.). (Antifung). Oral antifungal/antiyeast drug. 149

miconazole (Monistat) (Ob/Gyn). Topical antiyeast drug for vaginal infections. 115

MICRhoGAM (Ob/Gyn). Given to Rh negative mothers with Rh positive babies before 12 weeks of gestation to suppress Rh sensitization. 118

microgram (mcg). 44-45

Micro-K (Uro). Potassium supplement taken with diuretics. 58

Micronase (Endo). Oral antidiabetic drug. 110

Micronor (Ob/Gyn) Progesterone-only oral contraceptive. 114

Microsulfon (Antibio). Sulfonamide anti-infective drug. 140

Midamor (Uro). Potassium-sparing diuretic. 58

midazolam (Versed) (Anes). Intravenous drug for induction of general anesthesia. 159

Midol (Ob/Gyn). Over-the-counter drug for dysmenorrhea. 115

migraine headache, drugs for. 19, 138-139

milk of magnesia (M.O.M.) (GI). Antacid. 6, 65

milliequivalent (mEq). 46

milligram (mg). 44-45

milliliter (ml). 45

Milontin (Neuro). Used for absence seizures. 121

milrinone (Primacor) (Cardio). Investigational non-digitalis drug for congestive heart failure. 75

Miltown (Psych). Antianxiety drug. 128

minim. 6, 44

Minipress (Cardio). An alpha₁ blocker antihypertensive drug. 83

Minitran (Cardio). Antianginal drug. 77

Minizide (Cardio). Antihypertensive and diuretic combination drug. 84

Minocin (Antibio). Tetracycline-type antibiotic. 116-117, 144

minocycline (Minocin) (Antibio). Tetracycline-type antibiotic. 116-117, 144

Minodyl (Cardio). Vasodilator. 83

minor tranquilizers (Psych). Class of drugs used for anxiety. 126-128

minoxidil (Loniten, Minodyl) (Cardio). Vasodilator. 83

minoxidil (Rogaine) (Derm). Topical vasodilator for baldness. 56, 84

Miochol (Oph). Miotic drug for glaucoma. 104

Miostat (Oph). Miotic drug for glaucoma. 104

miotic (Oph). Class of drugs which constrict the pupil; used to treat glaucoma. 104-105

Miradon (Hem). Anticoagulant. 92

misoprostol (Cytotec) (GI). Used to prevent ulcers in patients on NSAIDs. 63, 73, 139

mites. 55

Mithracin (Chemo). Antibiotic used only for chemotherapy. 153

mitomycin (Mutamycin) (Chemo). Antibiotic used only for chemotherapy. 153

mitoxantrone (Novantrone) (Chemo). Antibiotic used only for chemotherapy. 153

Mitrolan (GI). Laxative. 65

Mixtard 70/30 (Endo). 70% NPH and 30% regular insulin. 110

ml (milliliter). 45

Moban (Psych). Antipsychotic drug. 129

Moctanin (GI). Used to dissolve gallstones. 68

Moderil (Cardio). Antihypertensive drug. 83

Moduretic (Uro). Potassium-wasting and potassium-sparing diuretic combination. 58

mold. 5, 15, 142

molindone (Moban) (Psych). Antipsychotic drug. 129

M.O.M. (milk of magnesia). (GI). Laxative. 65

monilia, infection with. 102, 148

Monistat (Ob/Gyn). Topical antiyeast drug for vaginal infections. 25, 115

Monistat i.v. (Antifung). Oral antifungal/antiyeast drug. 149

monoamine oxidase (MAO) inhibitors (Psych). Class of antidepressant drugs. 129-131

monobactams (Antibio). Class of antibiotics for gram-negative bacteria. 145

Monocid (Antibio). Cephalosporin antibiotic. 143

monoclonal antibody. 6

monoctanoin (Moctanin) (GI). Used to dissolve gallstones. 68

monophasic oral contraceptives (Ob/Gyn). 113

mood-elevating drugs. 129-133

morphine sulfate (Duramorph, MS Contin) (Analges). Narcotic analgesic drug. 5, 6, 8, 10, 135

moricizine (Ethmozine) (Cardio). Antiarrhythmic drug. 79

morning sickness. 9

Motilium (GI). Used for nausea after chemotherapy. 67

Motofen (GI). Narcotic antidiarrheal drug. 64

Motrin (Analges, Ob/Gyn, Ortho). Used to treat dysmenorrhea; nonsteroidal anti-inflammatory drug. 70, 115, 138

moxalactam (Moxam) (Antibio). Third-generation cephalosporin antibiotic. 143

Moxam (Antibio). Third-generation cephalosporin antibiotic. 143

MS Contin (Analgesic). Narcotic analgesic drug. 135

MTBE (GI). Used to dissolve gallstones. 68

Mucomyst (Resp). Mucus-thinning agent; antidote for Tylenol overdose. 96-97, 139

musculoskeletal drugs. 69-73

Mustargen (Chemo). Alkylating chemotherapy drug. 152

Mutamycin (Chemo). Antibiotic used only for chemotherapy. 153

Myambutol (Resp). Antitubercular drug. 96

Mycelex (Derm, ENT). Topical antifungal/antiyeast drug for mouth/skin. 54, 101

Mycelex-G (Ob/Gyn). Topical antiyeast drug for vaginal infection. 115

Mycifradin (GI). Oral antibiotic given before GI surgery to inhibit bacterial growth in the GI tract. 28, 68

Mycitracin Ophthalmic (Oph). Topical antibiotic combination for the eye. 103

Mycobacterium tuberculosis. 96

Mycolog (Derm). Topical anti-inflammatory/antifungal combination. 56

Mycostatin (ENT). Topical antifungal/antiyeast drug for mouth. 101

Mycostatin (Ob/Gyn). Topical antifungal/antiyeast drug for vaginal infection. 148

Mydriacyl (Oph). Mydriatic drug. 105

mydriatics (Oph). Class of drugs which dilate the pupil. 41, 105

Mylanta (GI). Antacid. 61

Myleran (Chemo). Alkylating chemotherapy drug. 152

Mylicon (GI). Antiflatulent. 62

Myochrysine (Ortho). Gold salts used for arthritis. 71

Mysoline (Neuro). Used to treat tonic-clonic seizures. 120-121

M.V.C. 9+3. Intravenous multivitamin complex with 12 vitamins. 163

M.V.I.-12. Intravenous multivitamin complex with 12 vitamins. 163

N, n

N₂O (Anes). Inhaled general anesthetic. 158, 160

nabilone (Cesamet) (GI). Used for nausea after chemotherapy. 67

nadolol (Corgard) (Cardio, Analges). Nonselective beta blocker drug used for angina and hypertension; also used for migraine headaches. 77, 79-80, 138

nafarelin (Synarel) (Ob/Gyn). Used to treat endometriosis. 112

nafcillin (Unipen) (Antibio). Penicillin-type antibiotic. 141

naftifine (Naftin) (Derm). Topical antifungal drug. 54

Naftin (Derm). Topical antifungal drug. 54

nalbuphine (Nubain) (Analges). Narcotic analgesic drug. 135

Naldecon (ENT). Decongestant with two antihistamines combination drug. 100

Nalfon (Ortho). Nonsteroidal anti-inflammatory drug. 70, 138

nalidixic (NegGram) (Uro). Urinary tract antibiotic. 59

naloxone (Narcan). Used to reverse narcotic overdose. 88, 139

names, drug. 13-15

Napa (Cardio). Investigational antiarrhythmic drug. 79

Naprosyn (Ob/Gyn, Ortho). Used to treat dysmenorrhea; nonsteroidal anti-inflammatory drug. 70, 115, 138

naproxen (Naprosyn) (Ob/Gyn, Ortho). Used to treat dysmenorrhea; nonsteroidal anti-inflammatory drug. 70, 115, 138

Narcan.Used to reverse narcotic overdose. 88, 139

narcotic (Analges). Class of addictive pain-killing drugs derived from opium. 64, 134, 137

Nardil (Psych). MAO inhibitor antidepressant. 131

Nasalcrom (ENT). Topical mast cell inhibitor for allergic rhinitis. 102

Nasalide (ENT). Intranasal corticosteroid. 101

National Formulary. 8

Naturetin (Uro). Thiazide diuretic. 57

Navane (Psych). Antipsychotic drug. 129

Nebcin (Antibio). Aminoglycoside antibiotic. 144

NebuPent (Resp). Used for *Pneumocystis carinii* infection. 147

nedocromil (Tilade) (Resp). Investigational mast cell inhibitor. 96

needle
bore of. 41
butterfly. 42
gauge of. 41

NegGram (Uro). Urinary tract antibiotic. 59

Nelova 10/11 (Ob/Gyn). Combination progesterone/estrogen oral contraceptive. 113

Nembutal (Sed/Hyp). Barbiturate drug for insomnia, sedation. 124

NeoDecadron (Oph). Topical corticosteroid/antibiotic combination. 104

neomycin (Derm). Topical antibiotic. 53

neomycin (Mycifradin) (GI). Oral antibiotic given before GI surgery to inhibit bacterial growth in GI tract. 28, 68

Neosporin Ophthalmic (Oph). Topical antibiotics combination for eye. 103

Neosporin (Derm). Topical antibiotic combination. 53

Neo-Synephrine (ENT). Decongestant. 98

Neotrizine (Uro). Sulfonamide anti-infective drug. 59

nephrotoxicity. 34, 144

Nesacaine (Anes). Local/regional anesthetic. 158-159

netilmicin (Netromycin) (Antibio). Aminoglycoside antibiotic. 144

Netromycin (Antibio). Aminoglycoside antibiotic. 144

neuroleptics (Psych). Major tranquilizers for psychosis. 128

neurological drugs. 119-125

neuromuscular blocking drug (Anes). Class of drugs which produce muscle relaxation during surgery. 160

neurosis, drugs for. 6, 126-128

neurotransmitter. 19, 36, 64, 129

niacin (nicotinic acid) (Cardio). Used for hyperlipidemia. 86

nicardipine (Cardene) (Cardio). Calcium channel blocking drug for angina and hypertension. 78, 82

Nicolar (Cardio). For hyperlipidemia. 86

nicotinic acid (Cardio). For hyperlipidemia. 86

nifedipine (Adalat, Procardia) (Cardio, Analges). Calcium channel blocking drug used for angina and hypertension. 78, 82

Nilstat (ENT). Topical antifungal/yeast drug for mouth. 101

Nilstat (Ob/Gyn). Topical antifungal/antiyeast drug for vaginal infection. 115

nimodipine (Nimotop) (Analges, Neuro). Calcium channel blocker used for migraine headaches and improved circulation after stroke. 139

Nimotop (Analges, Neuro). Calcium channel blocker for migraine headaches and improved circulation after stroke. 139

Nipride (Cardio). For hypertensive crisis. 82

nitrates (Cardio). Class of antianginal drugs. 76-77

nitrendipine (Baypress) (Cardio). Investigational calcium channel blocker. 82

Nitro-Bid (Cardio). Antianginal drug. 77

Nitrocap T. D. (Cardio). Antianginal drug. 77

Nitrodisc (Cardio). Antianginal drug. 77

Nitro-Dur (Cardio). Antianginal drug. 77

nitrofurantoin (Furadantin, Macrodantin) (Uro). Urinary tract antibiotic. 59

nitrofurazone (Furacin) (Derm). Topical antibiotic for burns. 56

Nitrogard (Cardio). Antianginal drug. 77

nitrogen mustard (Chemo). Alkylating chemotherapy drug. 67, 152

nitroglycerin (Nitro-Bid, Nitro-Dur) (Cardio). Antianginal drug. 76-77

nitroglycerin ointment. 22, 45-46, 77

nitroglycerin spray. 22, 76

nitroglycerin, sublingual. 24, 76

Nitrol (Cardio). Antianginal drug. 77

Nitrolingual (Cardio). Antianginal drug. 77

Nitrong (Cardio). Antianginal drug. 77

nitroprusside (Nipride) (Cardio). For hypertensive crisis. 82

Nitrospan (Cardio). Antianginal drug. 77

Nitrostat (Cardio). Antianginal drug. 77

nitrous oxide (N_2O) (Anes). Inhaled general anesthetic. 25, 157, 160

Nitro-Bid (Cardio). Antianginal drug. 77

Nitro-Dur (Cardio). Antianginal drug. 77

nits. 55

Nix (Derm). Topical drug for pediculosis or lice. 55

nizatidine (Axid) (GI). H_2 blocker to heal ulcers. 62

Nizoral (Antifung). Topical and oral antifungal/antiyeast drug. 54, 149

Noctec (Sed/Hyp). Nonbarbiturate nighttime sedative. 29, 123

Noludar (Sed/Hyp). Nonbarbiturate drug for short-term insomnia. 124

Nolvadex (Chemo). Hormonal chemotherapy drug. 153

nonselective beta blockers (Cardio). 80

nonsteroidal anti-inflammatory drugs (NSAID) (Analges, Ortho). Class of drugs that reduce pain and inflammation. 70, 138

Norcuron (Anes). Neuromuscular blocking drug. 160

norepinephrine (Levophed) (Cardio). Vasopressor for hypotension. 90

norepinephrine (neurotransmitter). 36, 129, 131

norethindrone (Aygestin, Norlutin) (Ob/Gyn). Used to treat amenorrhea. 114

Norflex (Ortho). Skeletal muscle relaxant. 72

norfloxacin (Noroxin) (Uro). Urinary tract antibiotic. 59

Norgesic (Ortho). Skeletal muscle relaxant and analgesic combination. 72

Norinyl 1+35 (Ob/Gyn). Combination progesterone/estrogen oral contraceptive. 113

Norinyl 1+50 (Ob/Gyn). Combination progesterone/estrogen oral contraceptive. 113

Norlestrin 1/50 (Ob/Gyn). Combination progesterone/estrogen oral contraceptive. 113

Norlestrin 2.5/50 (Ob/Gyn). Combination progesterone/estrogen oral contraceptive. 113

Norlutate (Ob/Gyn). Used to treat amenorrhea. 114

Norlutin (Ob/Gyn). Used to treat amenorrhea. 114

normal saline (NS). Intravenous fluids of 0.9% NaCl. 163

Normodyne (Cardio). Alpha and beta blocker drug used for hypertension. 80

Noroxin (Uro). Urinary tract antibiotic. 59

Norpace (Cardio). Antiarrhythmic drug. 79

Norplant (Ob/Gyn). Progesterone-only intradermal implant contraceptive. 114

Norpramin (Psych). Tricyclic antidepressant. 131

nortriptyline (Aventyl, Pamelor) (Psych). Tricyclic antidepressant. 131

Novahistine (ENT). Decongestant and antihistamine combination. 100

Novantrone (Chemo). Antibiotic used only for chemotherapy. 153

Novapren (Antivir). AIDS drug. 146

novobiocin (Albamycin) (Antibio). Antibiotic. 145

Novocain (Anes). Local/regional/spinal anesthetic. 157-159

Novolin L (Endo). Injectable lente insulin. 109

Novolin N (Endo). Injectable NPH insulin. 109

Novolin R (Endo). Injectable regular insulin. 109

Novolin 70/30 (Endo). 70% NPH and 30% regular insulin, injectable. 110

NPH Iletin (Endo). Injectable NPH insulin. 109

NPH insulin (NPH Iletin, Humulin N) (Endo). Injectable NPH insulin. 109

n.p.o. (nothing by mouth).

NS. Abbreviation for *normal saline* intravenous fluid. 163

NSAID (Ortho). Abbreviation for nonsteroidal anti-inflammatory drug. 9, 61, 63, 70-72, 138

Nubain (Analges). Narcotic analgesic drug. 135

Numorphan (Analges). Narcotic analgesic drug. 135

Nupercainal (Derm). Topical anesthetic drug. 158

Nuprin (Analges, Ob/Gyn, Ortho). Nonsteroidal, anti-inflammatory drug. 70, 138

NutriLipid. Intravenous fat solution. 163

Nydrazid (Resp). Antitubercular drug. 96

nylidrin (Arlidin) (Cardio). Peripheral vasodilating drug. 84

NyQuil (ENT). Decongestant, antitussive, pain reliever combination drug. 100

nystatin (Mycostatin, Nilstat) (ENT, Ob/Gyn). Topical antifungal/antiyeast for mouth and for vaginal infections. 101, 115-116, 148

Nytol (Sed/Hyp). Over-the-counter nonbarbiturate drug for insomnia. 124

■

O, o

oxycodone (Roxicodone) (Analges). Narcotic analgesic drug. 135

oxiconazole (Oxistat) (Derm). Topical antifungal drug. 54

Oxistat (Derm). Topical antifungal drug. 54

Oxsoralen (Derm). For severe, disabling psoriasis. 52

oxtriphylline (Choledyl) (Resp). Bronchodilator. 95

Oxy 5 (Derm). Topical acne drug. 51

oxymetazoline (Afrin, Duration) (ENT). Decongestant. 98

oxymorphone (Numorphan) (Analges). Narcotic analgesic drug. 135

oxyphencyclimine (Daricon) (GI). Antispasmodic drug. 64

oxytetracycline (Terramycin) (Antibio, Derm). Oral, I.M., and topical antibiotic. 53, 144

oxytocin (Pitocin) (Ob/Gyn). Stimulates uterine contractions. 112

P, p

packed red blood cells (PRBC) (Hem). RBCs without plasma. 163

Pamelor (Psych). Tricyclic antidepressant. 131

Pamine (GI). Antispasmodic drug. 64

Pamprin (Ob/Gyn). Over-the-counter drug for dysmenorrhea. 115

Panadol (Analges). Nonaspirin analgesic drug. 137

Pancrease (GI). Pancreatic digestive enzyme supplement. 68

pancrelipase (Cotazym) (GI). Pancreatic digestive enzyme supplement. 68

pancuronium (Pavulon) (Anes). Intraoperative muscle-paralyzing drug. 160

Pantopon (Analges). Narcotic analgesic drug. 135

Paradione (Neuro). Used to treat absence seizures. 121

Parafon Forte DSC (Ortho). Skeletal muscle relaxant. 72

paraldehyde (Sed/Hyp). For sedation during alcohol withdrawal. 125

paramethadione (Paradione) (Neuro). Used to treat absence seizures. 121

paramethasone (Haldrone) (Endo). Oral anti-inflammatory drug. 108

Paraplatin (Chemo). Chemotherapy drug. 152

paregoric (GI). Narcotic antidiarrheal drug. 6, 10, 64

parenteral administration. 25-27

Parkinson disease, drugs for. 6, 29, 118, 121-123

Parlodel (Neuro). Used to treat Parkinson disease. 122-123

Parlodel (Ob/Gyn). Inhibits postpartum milk production. 117-118

Parnate (Psych). MAO inhibitor antidepressant. 131

Parsidol (Neuro). Used to treat Parkinson disease. 123

patch, transdermal. 23, 77, 114

patent ductus arteriosus, drugs for. 19

patent medicines. 8

patent on new drugs. 19-20

Pathocil (Antibio). Penicillin-type antibiotic. 141

pathogen. 42

Pavulon (Anes). Intraoperative muscle-paralyzing drug. 160

Paxarel (Sed/Hyp). Nonbarbiturate daytime sedative.

Paxipam (Psych). Benzodiazepine antianxiety drug. 13, 127

p.c. (after meals).

PCP (phencyclidine). An illicit drug. 10

peak level of drug. 42

Pedialyte. Oral electrolyte solution for infants.

Pediamycin (Antibio). Erythromycin antibiotic. 145

pediatric patients. 23, 30, 47-48

Pediazole (Antibio). Erythromycin and sulfonamide anti-infective combination drug. 145

pediculosis, drugs for. 55

Peganone (Neuro). Used for tonic-clonic seizures. 120-121

pelvic inflammatory disease, drugs for. 116

pemoline (Cylert) (Neuro). For attention deficit disorder, a CNS stimulant. 124

penbutolol (Levatol) (Cardio). Nonselective beta blocking drug used for hypertension. 80

penicillin. 5-6, 18, 35, 45, 141-143

penicillinase. 141

penicillin G (Antibio). Antibiotic. 15, 86, 141

penicillin G benzathine (Bicillin, Permapen) (Antibio). Antibiotic. 141

penicillin G potassium (Pentids) (Antibio). Antibiotic. 117, 141

penicillin G procaine (Duracillin, Wycillin) (Antibio). Antibiotic. 116-117, 141

penicillin V (Pen-Vee K, V-Cillin K) (Antibio). Antibiotic. 116-117, 141

Penicillium chrysogenum. 15, 142

pentaerythritol tetranitrate (Peritrate) (Cardio). Antianginal drug. 77

Pentam 300 (Resp). For *Pneumocystis carinii* infection. 147

pentamidine (NebuPent) (Resp). For *Pneumocystis carinii* infection. 147

pentamidine (Pentam 300) (Resp). For *Pneumocystis carinii* infection. 147

pentazocine (Talwin) (Analges). Narcotic analgesic drug. 135

Penthrane (Anes). Inhaled general anesthetic. 160

Pentids (Antibio). Penicillin-type antibiotic. 116, 141

pentobarbital (Nembutal) (Sed/Hyp). Barbiturate drug for sedation, insomnia. 124

Pentothal (Anes). Intravenous barbiturate for induction of general anesthesia. 26, 157, 159

pentoxifylline (Trental) (Cardio). Decreases blood viscosity to improve flow. 86

Pen-Vee K (Antibio). Penicillin-type antibiotic. 116, 141

Pepcid (GI). H₂ blocker to heal ulcers.

peptic ulcer disease. 6, 61

percentage (drug measurement). 46

Percocet (Analges). Narcotic analgesic. 137

Percodan (Analges). Narcotic analgesic. 137

Percogesic (ENT). Antihistamine and pain reliever combination drug. 100

Percorten (Endo). Used to treat Addison disease. 108

Perdiem (GI). Laxative. 65

pergolide mesylate (Permax) (Neuro). Used to treat Parkinson disease. 122

Pergonal (Ob/Gyn). Ovulation-stimulating drug for infertility. 111

Periactin (Derm). Oral antipruritic drug. 54

Peritrate (Cardio). Antianginal drug. 77

periwinkle (plant). 5, 153

Permapen (Antibio). Penicillin-type antibiotic. 141

Permax (Neuro). Used to treat Parkinson disease. 122

permethrin (Nix) (Derm). Topical drug for pediculosis or lice. 55

pernicious anemia. 26, 68, 87

perphenazine (Trilafon) (Psych, GI). Phenothiazine antipsychotic drug; antiemetic. 66-67, 129

Persantine (Cardio, Hem). Used in thallium testing; anticoagulant. 86, 92

Pertussin (ENT). Nonnarcotic antitussive. 99-100

P.E.T.N. (Cardio). Antianginal drug. 77

pharmacodynamics. 1

pharmacology
ancient. 3-5
definition of. 1
history of. 3-7
molecular. 1

Phazyme (GI). Antiflatulent. 62

phenacemide (Phenurone) (Neuro). Anticonvulsant. 121

phenazopyridine (Pyridium, Urogesic) (Uro). Urinary tract analgesic. 59

phenelzine (Nardil) (Psych). MAO inhibitor antidepressant. 131

Phenergan (GI). Antiemetic. 66-67

Phenergan With Codeine. Antihistamine and narcotic antitussive combination drug. 100

phenobarbital (Luminal) (Neuro). Used for tonic-clonic seizures. 6, 10, 120-121

phenothiazine derivative (Psych). Class of drugs used to treat psychosis. 129

Phenurone (Neuro). Anticonvulsant. 121

phensuximide (Milontin) (Neuro). Used for absence seizures. 121

phenylbutazone (Butazolidin) (Ortho). Anti-inflammatory drug. 71-72

phenylephrine (Neo-Synephrine) (ENT). Decongestant. 98

phenylpropanolamine (ENT). Decongestant. 98

phenytoin (Dilantin) (Neuro). Used for tonic-clonic seizures. 20, 120-121

Phillips' Milk of Magnesia (GI). Laxative. 65

pHisoHex (Derm). Topical antibacterial scrub. 56

phocomelia. 9

physostigmine (Oph). Miotic drug for glaucoma. 105

Pilagan (Oph). Miotic drug for glaucoma. 104

Pilocar (Oph). Miotic drug for glaucoma. 104

pilocarpine (Ocusert Pilo, Pilagan, Pilocar) (Oph). Miotic drug for glaucoma. 104

pinacidil (Pindac) (Cardio). Investigational vasodilator. 83

Pindac (Cardio). Investigational vasodilator. 83

pindolol (Visken) (Cardio). Nonselective beta blocker drug used to treat hypertension. 79-80

piperacillin (Pipracil) (Antibio). Penicillin-type antibiotic. 116, 141

pipobroman (Vercyte) (Chemo). Chemotherapy drug. 152

Pipracil (Antibio). Penicillin-type antibiotic. 116, 141

pirbuterol (Maxair) (Resp). Bronchodilator. 94

pirenzepine (Gastrozepine) (GI). Investigational antiulcer drug. 63

piroxicam (Feldene) (Ortho). Nonsteroidal anti-inflammatory drug. 70, 138

Pitocin (Ob/Gyn). Stimulates uterine contractions. 112

Pitressin (Endo). Used to treat diabetes insipidus. 108

placebo. 42

placenta. 29

Placidyl (Sed/Hyp). Nonbarbiturate drug for insomnia. 123

Plasbumin-5 (Hem). Albumin 5% given intravenously to increase blood volume. 165

Plasbumin-25 (Hem). Albumin 25% given intravenously to increase blood volume. 165

plasma protein fraction (PPF) (Hem). Given intravenously to increase blood volume. 165

plasma protein fraction (Plasmanate) (Hem). Given intravenously to increase blood volume. 165

plasma proteins. 29-30

plasma volume expanders (Hem). Given intravenously to increase blood volume.

Plasmanate (Hem). Plasma protein fraction given intravenously to increase blood volume. 165

Plasma-Plex (Hem). Plasma protein given intravenously to increase blood volume. 165

Plasmatein (Hem). Plasma protein fraction given intravenously to increase blood volume. 165

Platinol (Chemo). Alkylating chemotherapy drug. 67, 152

plicamycin (Mithracin) (Chemo). Antibiotic used only for chemotherapy. 153

PMB (Ob/Gyn). Estrogen and antianxiety combination drug for menopause. 114

Pneumocystis carinii. 146-147

p.o., PO (per os, by mouth).

Polycillin (Antibio). Penicillin-type antibiotic. 19, 116, 141

polyestradiol (Estradurin) (Chemo). Hormonal chemotherapy drug. 153

polymyxin B (Antibio). Topical antibiotic. 53

Polysporin (Derm, Oph). Topical and ophthalmic antibiotic combination drug. 53, 103

polythiazide (Renese) (Uro). Thiazide diuretic. 57

Ponstel (Ob/Gyn). Used to treat dysmenorrhea. 115

Pontocaine (Anes). Spinal/epidural anesthetic. 159

Pontocaine (Derm, Oph). Topical and ophthalmic anesthetic. 104, 158

Potage (Uro). Potassium supplement taken with diuretics. 58

potassium clavulanate (Antibio). Used with ticarcillin to keep it from being broken down by penicillinase. 145

potassium-sparing diuretic (Uro). Class of diuretics which cause less potassium than usual to be lost in the urine. 58

potassium supplements (Kay Ciel, K-Dur, Slow-K) (Uro). Class of drugs given with diuretics to replace lost potassium. 14, 46, 58

potassium-wasting diuretics (Uro). Class of diuretics which cause potassium to be lost in the urine. 58

PPF (plasma protein fraction) (Hem). Given intravenously to increase blood volume. 165

pramoxine (Tronothane) (Derm). Topical anesthetic drug. 158

prazepam (Centrax) (Psych). Benzodiazepine antianxiety drug. 13, 128

prazosin (Minipress) (Cardio). An alpha$_1$ blocker drug for hypertension. 83

PRBC (Hem). Red blood cells without plasma. 164

Precef (Antibio). Second-generation cephalosporin antibiotic. 116, 143

Pred Forte (Oph). Topical corticosteroid for eye. 104

prednisolone (Delta-Cortef) (Endo, Ortho). Oral corticosteroid anti-inflammatory drug. 71, 108

prednisolone (Inflamase, Pred Forte) (Oph). Topical corticosteroid for eye. 71, 108

prednisone (Deltasone) (Endo, Ortho). Oral corticosteroid anti-inflammatory drug. 71, 108

Pregnyl (Ob/Gyn). Ovulation-stimulating drug for infertility. 111

preload (Cardio). 76

Premarin (Ob/Gyn). Estrogen replacement for menopause. 14, 25, 114

premature baby. See *pediatric patients.*

prescription, definition of. 3

prescription drugs. 11, 49

prescription form. 49

Primacor (Cardio). Investigational nondigitalis drug for congestive heart failure. 75

Primatene Mist (Resp). Over-the-counter bronchodilator. 22, 94-95

Primaxin (Antibio). Antibiotic. 145

primidone (Mysoline) (Neuro). Used to treat tonic-clonic seizures. 120-121

Principen (Antibio). Penicillin-type antibiotic. 19, 141

Prinivil (Cardio). ACE inhibitor drug used for hypertension. 82

Priscoline (Cardio). For pulmonary hypertension in newborns. 86

p.r.n. (pro re nata, as needed).

Pro-Banthine (GI). Antispasmodic. 64

probenecid (Antibio). Prolongs levels of ampicillin in blood. 145

probenecid (Benemid) (Ortho). Used for gout. 72

probucol (Lorelco) (Cardio). Used for hypercholesterolemia. 85

procainamide (Procan SR, Pronestyl) (Cardio). Antiarrhythmic drug. 79

procaine (Novocain) (Anes). Local/regional/spinal anesthetic. 157-159

Procan SR (Cardio). Antiarrhythmic drug. 21, 79

procarbazine (Matulane) (Chemo). Chemotherapy drug. 155

Procardia (Cardio). Calcium channel blocking agent for angina and hypertension. 78, 82

prochlorperazine (Compazine) (GI). Antiemetic. 66-67

procyclidine (Kemadrin) (Neuro). Used to treat Parkinson disease. 123

Progestasert (Ob/Gyn). Progesterone-only uterine contraceptive. 114

progesterone. 113-114

Prolixin (Psych). Phenothiazine antipsychotic drug. 129

Proloid (Endo). Thyroid hormone replacement. 107

promazine (Sparine) (Psych). Phenothiazine antipsychotic drug. 129

Promega (Cardio). Used for hyperlipidemia. 86

promethazine (Phenergan) (GI). Antiemetic. 66-67

Pronestyl (Cardio). Antiarrhythmic drug. 79

Propa P.H. (Derm). Topical acne preparation. 51

propafenone (Rythmol) (Cardio). Antiarrhythmic drug. 79

propantheline (Pro-Banthine) (GI). Used for peptic ulcer; antispasmodic. 64

proparacaine (Ophthaine) (Oph). Topical anesthetic for eye. 104

prophylactic. 42

Propine (Oph). Miotic drug for glaucoma. 105

propoxyphene (Darvon) (Analges). Narcotic analgesic drug. 135

propranolol (Inderal) (Cardio, Analges). Nonselective beta blocking drug used to treat hypertension, arrhythmias, angina; migraine headaches. 19, 77, 79-80, 139 propylthiouracil (Endo). Used to treat hyperthyroidism. 107

ProSom (Neuro, Sed/Hyp). Investigational nonbarbiturate drug for insomnia. 123

prostaglandin. 69-70

prostaglandin E1 (Cardio). See *alprostadil*. 86, 115

Prostaphlin (Antibio). Penicillin-type antibiotic. 141

Prostin E2 (Ob/Gyn). Prostaglandin used to abort fetus. 115

Prostin F2 Alpha (Ob/Gyn). Prostaglandin used to abort fetus. 115

Prostin VR (Cardio). Used to keep open ductus arteriosus in newborn infants with congenital heart disease. 86, 115

protamine sulfate (Hem). Reverses effects of heparin. 93

protamine zinc (PZI) (Endo). Injectable insulin.

Prothiaden (Psych). Investigational tricyclic antidepressant. 131

Proto-Chol (Cardio). Used for hyperlipidemia. 86

prototype. 42

protriptyline (Vivactil) (Psych). Tricyclic antidepressant. 131

Protropin (Endo). Growth hormone replacement. 107

Proventil (Resp). Bronchodilator. 25, 94

Provera (Ob/Gyn). Used to treat amenorrhea. 114

Prozac (Psych). Antidepressant. 131

pseudoephedrine (Afrinol, Sudafed) (ENT). Decongestant. 14, 98

psoralens (Derm). Class of drugs used for severe psoriasis. 52

psoriasis, drugs for. 52

psychiatric drugs. 126-133

psychosis. 6, 128-129

pulmonary drugs. 94-97

purine antagonist (Chemo). Class of chemotherapy drugs. 151

Purinethol (Chemo). Purine antagonist chemotherapy drug. 151

PUVA (Derm). Abbreviation for psoralen/ ultraviolet wavelength A. 52

Pyopen (Antibio). Penicillin-type antibiotic. 116, 141

pyrazinamide (Resp). Antituberculosis drug. 96

Pyridium (Uro). Urinary tract analgesic. 59

Pyridium Plus (Uro). Urinary analgesic, antispasmodic and sedative. 59

pyrimidine antagonist (Chemo). Class of chemotherapy drugs. 151

PZI (protamine zinc) (Endo). Injectable insulin. 109

Q, q

q.d. (every day).
q.h. (every hour).
q.h.s. (at every bedtime).
q.i.d. (four times a day).
q.o.d. (every other day).
Quarzan (GI). Antispasmodic drug. 64
quazepam (Doral) (Sed/Hyp). Nonbarbiturate benzodiazepine for insomnia. 124
Questran (Cardio). Used for hypercholesterolemia. 85
Quibron (Resp). Bronchodilator. 95

Quinaglute (Cardio). Antiarrhythmic drug. 79
quinestrol (Estrovis) (Ob/Gyn). Estrogen replacement for menopause. 114
quinethazone (Hydromox) (Uro). Thiazide diuretic. 57
Quinidex (Cardio). Antiarrhythmic drug. 79
quinidine (Cardioquin, Quinaglute) (Cardio). Antiarrhythmic drug. 79
quinine. 5

■

R, r

R & C (Derm). Topical drug for pediculosis or lice. 55

racemic. 42

radioactive sodium iodide 131 (Endo). Used to treat hyperthyroidism. 107

ranitidine (Zantac) (GI). H_2 blocker to heal ulcers. 62

ratio (drug measurement). 46

Rauwolfia serpentina (plant). 5

receptor 16, 35
    adrenergic. 36, 38, 83
    alpha. 36, 83, 138
    beta$_1$ and beta$_2$. 36, 81, 138
    cholinergic. 36, 39, 64
    H_1. 36, 63, 99
    H_2. 36, 62-63

recombinant DNA. 6

rectal administration of drugs. 25, 28

Reglan (GI). Gastric stimulant. 66-67

Regular Iletin (Endo). Injectable regular insulin. 109

regular insulin (Regular Iletin, Humulin R) (Endo). Injectable regular insulin. 109

Renese (Uro). Thiazide diuretic. 57

Renese-R (Cardio). Antihypertensive and diuretic combination drug.

Renoquid (Antibio). Sulfonamide anti-infective drug. 59

Repetab. Part of trade name of drug, indicating a sustained-release tablet. 42

rescinnamine (Moderil) (Cardio). Antihypertensive drug. 83

reserpine (Serpasil) (Cardio). Antihypertensive drug. 5, 83

Respbid (Resp). Bronchodilator. 95

Respihaler (Resp). Inhaled corticosteroid.

respiratory drugs. 94-97

Restoril (Sed/Hyp). Nonbarbiturate benzodiazepine drug for insomnia. 124

resuscitation, emergency drugs for. 27, 88-91

Retin-A (Derm). Topical drug for acne and skin wrinkles. 52, 56

Retrovir (Antivir). AIDS drug. 146

Reye syndrome. 136

Rheomacrodex (Hem). Plasma volume expander. 165

Rheumatrex (Ortho). For rheumatoid arthritis. 71

RhoGAM (Ob/Gyn). Given to Rh negative mothers with Rh positive baby after delivery to suppress Rh sensitization. 118

ribavirin (Virazole) (Antivir). Used for herpes simplex virus; AIDS drug; also for respiratory syncytial virus. 146, 148

RID (Derm). Topical drug for pediculosis or lice. 55

Ridaura (Ortho). Gold salts used for arthritis. 71

Rifabutin (Antivir). AIDS drug. 146

Rifadin (Resp). Antitubercular drug. 96

rifampin (Rifadin, Rimactane) (Resp). Antitubercular drug. 96

Rimactane (Resp). Antitubercular drug. 96

Rimadyl (Ortho). Investigational nonsteroidal anti-inflammatory drug. 70, 138

rimantadine (Flumadine) (Antivir). For influenza virus A. 148

Ringer's lactate (RL). Intravenous fluid of dextrose, electrolytes, and normal saline. 163

Riopan (GI). Antacid. 61

Ritalin (Neuro). Used for attention deficit disorder, a CNS stimulant. 124

ritodrine (Yutopar) (Ob/Gyn). Used to stop premature labor contractions. 112

RL (Ringer's lactate). Intravenous fluid of dextrose, electrolytes, and normal saline. 163

Robaxin (Ortho). Skeletal muscle relaxant. 72

Robaxisal (Ortho). Skeletal muscle relaxant and analgesic combination drug. 72

Robinul (GI). Antispasmodic drug. 64

Robitussin (ENT). Expectorant. 99

Rocaltrol (Ortho). Used to increase bone absorption of calcium for osteoporosis. 72

Rocephin (Antibio). Cephalosporin antibiotic. 116, 143

Roferon-A (Antivir, Chemo). AIDS and chemotherapy drug. 146, 155

Rogaine (Derm). Topical vasodilator for male-pattern baldness. 56, 84

Rolaids (GI). Antacid. 62

Roman numerals. 46-47

Rondec (ENT). Decongestant and antihistamine combination drug. 100

Rondomycin (Antibio). Tetracycline-type antibiotic. 116-117, 144

rose hips (plant). 5

Rowasa (GI). Topical anti-inflammatory for ulcerative colitis. 65

Roxicodone (Analges). Narcotic analgesic drug. 135

Robinul (GI). Antispasmodic drug. 64

routes of administration. 23-27, 50

Rubrex (Chemo). Antibiotic used only for chemotherapy. 153

Rufen (Analges, Ob/Gyn, Ortho). Used for dysmenorrhea; nonsteroidal anti-inflammatory drug. 70, 138

Rx, definition of. 3, 49

Rythmol (Cardio). Antiarrhythmic drug. 14-15, 79

■

S, s

s̄ *(sine)*, without.

SA (abbreviation for *sustained action*). Part of trade name of drug.

salicylates (Analges). Class of aspirin and related anti-inflammatory drugs. 69-70, 135

Saluron (Uro). Thiazide diuretic. 57

Sandostatin (GI). For severe diarrhea from cancerous GI tumor. 68

Sansert (Analges). Used for migraine headaches. 138

scabies. 55

schedule drug. 10-11, 49

sclerosing agents. 68

scopolamine (GI, Oph). Used for motion sickness; mydriatic drug. 3-4, 67, 105

scruple. 6, 44

"seal limbs." 9

secobarbital (Seconal) (Sed/Hyp). Barbiturate drug for insomnia. 124

Seconal (Sed/Hyp). Barbiturate drug for insomnia. 124

Sectral (Cardio). Cardioselective beta blocker drug used to treat hypertension and arrhythmias. 79, 81

sedative/hypnotics (Psych). Class of drugs used to produce sedation and sleep; may be barbiturates or nonbarbiturates. 123-124

seizures. See *epilepsy.*

Seldane (ENT). Antihistamine. 15, 99

selective beta blockers (Cardio). 81

selegiline (Eldepryl) (Neuro). Used to treat Parkinson disease. 122

Semilente Iletin (Endo). Injectable semilente insulin. 109

semilente insulin (Semilente Iletin) (Endo). Injectable semilente insulin. 109

Senokot (GI). Laxative. 65

Septra (Antibio). Antibiotic and sulfonamide anti-infective combination drug. 145

Sequels. Part of trade name of drug, indicating a slow-release capsule. 42

Ser-Ap-Es (Cardio). Combination antihypertensive and diuretic. 14, 84

Serax (Psych). Benzodiazepine antianxiety drug. 13, 128

Serentil (Psych). Phenothiazine antipsychotic drug. 129

serotonin (neurotransmitter). 129, 138

Serpasil (Cardio). Antihypertensive drug. 5, 14, 83

sexually transmitted disease (STD). 104, 116-117

sheep's wool. 5

side effect. 33-34

Silvadene (Derm). Topical antibacterial for burns. 56

silver nitrate (ENT). Cautery for stopping nosebleeds. 56, 102

silver nitrate (Oph). Used to prevent blindness in newborns caused by gonorrhea. 103-104, 117

silver sulfadiazine (Silvadene) (Derm). Topical antibacterial for burns. 56

simethicone (GI). Antiflatulent. 62

Sinemet (Neuro). Used for Parkinson disease. 123

Sinequan (Psych). Tricyclic antidepressant with antianxiety effect. 128, 131

Sine-Aid (ENT). Decongestant and pain reliever combination drug. 100

Skelaxin (Ortho). Skeletal muscle relaxant. 72

skeletal muscle relaxants (Ortho). Class of drugs used to prevent muscular spasm and tightness. 72

SL (sublingual).

sleep aids, sleeping pills. 33, 123-124

Slow-K (Uro). Potassium supplement given with diuretics. 14, 58

Slo-bid (Resp). Bronchodilator. 95

Slo-Phyllin Gyrocaps (Resp). Bronchodilator. 95

SMX (sulfamethoxazole). 144

snakeroot (plant). 5

sodium bicarbonate (Emerg, GI). Emergency drug; antacid. 62, 90

sodium hyaluronate (Amvisc, Healon) (Oph). Aqueous humor replacement. 106

sodium iodide 131, radioactive (Endo). Used to treat hyperthyroidism. 107

sodium pentothal. See *Pentothal*.

Solarcaine (Derm). Over-the-counter topical anesthetic. 158

Solganal (Ortho). Gold salts used for arthritis. 71

Solu-Cortef (Endo, Ortho). Oral corticosteroid anti-inflammatory drug. 71, 108

Solu-Medrol (Endo, Ortho). Oral corticosteroid anti-inflammatory drug. 71, 108

Soma (Ortho). Skeletal muscle relaxant. 72

Soma Compound (Ortho). Skeletal muscle relaxant and analgesic combination drug. 72

somatrem (Protropin) (Endo). Growth hormone replacement. 107

somatropin (Humatrope) (Endo). Growth hormone replacement. 107

Sominex (Sed/Hyp). Over-the-counter nonbarbiturate drug for insomnia. 124

Somophyllin (Resp). Bronchodilator. 94-95

Sorbitrate (Cardio). Antianginal drug. 77

sources of drugs. 15-17

Spansule. Part of trade name of drug, indicating a slow-release capsule. 42

Sparine (Psych). Phenothiazine antipsychotic drug. 129

Spectazole (Derm). Topical antifungal drug. 54

spectinomycin (Antibio). Oral antibiotic. 117

Spectrobid (Antibio). Penicillin-type antibiotic. 14, 116, 141

spelling drug names. 13-14

Spinhaler turbo-inhaler. 95

spironolactone (Aldactone) (Uro). Potassium-sparing diuretic. 58

Sprinkle. Part of trade name of drug, indicating that a capsule can be opened and the contents sprinkled on food to be administered. 43

SQ (subcutaneous).

SR (slow release). Part of trade name of drug. 21, 43

Stadol (Analges). Non-narcotic analgesic drug. 135

Staphcillin (Antibio). Penicillin-type antibiotic. 141

"Starry Night, The" (painting). 76

Staticin (Derm). Topical antiacne drug. 51

STD (sexually transmitted diseases). 104, 116-117

Stelazine (Psych). Phenothiazine antipsychotic drug. 129

step-care approach. 80

steroid. See *corticosteroid*.

Stilphostrol (Chemo). Hormonal chemotherapy drug. 153

stimulant, CNS (Neuro). Class of drugs used to treat attention deficit disorder. 124

stimulant, gastric (GI). 66

stool softener. 65

Streptase (Cardio, Hem). Thrombolytic enzyme. 92

streptokinase (Kabikinase, Streptase) (Cardio, Hem). Thrombolytic enzyme. 92

streptomycin. 15, 96

streptozocin (Zanosar) (Chemo). Alkylating chemotherapy drug. 152

Stri-Dex (Derm). Topical acne drug. 51

subcu (subcutaneous).

subcutaneous administration. 25-26, 28

Sublimaze (Anes). Intravenous general anesthetic. 160

sublingual administration. 24, 76

subQ (subcutaneous).

succinylcholine (Anectine, Sucostrin) (Anes). Intraoperative muscle-paralyzing drug. 160

Sucostrin (Anes). Intraoperative muscle-paralyzing agent. 160

sucralfate (Carafate) (GI). Antiulcer drug. 63

Sucrets (ENT). Non-narcotic antitussive. 99

Sudafed (ENT). Decongestant. 14, 25, 98

Sufenta (Anes). Intravenous general anesthetic. 160

sufentanil (Sufenta) (Anes). Intravenous general anesthetic. 160

sulconazole (Exelderm) (Derm). Topical antifungal drug. 54

sulfacytine (Renoquid) (Antibio). Sulfonamide anti-infective drug. 59, 140

sulfadiazine (Microsulfon) (Antibio). Sulfonamide anti-infective drug. 140

sulfa drugs. 140. See also *sulfonamides*.

sulfamethizole (Thiosulfil) (Uro). Sulfonamide anti-infective drug. 59, 140

sulfamethoxazole (Gantanol, SMX) (Uro). Sulfonamide anti-infective drug. 59, 140, 144

Sulfamylon (Derm). Topical antibacterial for burns. 56

sulfanilamide (AVC) (Ob/Gyn). Topical sulfa drug for vaginal yeast infection. 6, 115, 140

sulfasalazine (Azulfidine) (Antibio). Sulfonamide anti-infective for ulcerative colitis. 66, 140

sulfinpyrazone (Anturane) (Ortho). Used for gout. 72

sulfisoxazole (Gantrisin) (Uro). Sulfonamide anti-infective. 59, 140

sulfonamides (Uro). Class of anti-infective drugs. 59, 140

sulindac (Clinoril) (Ortho). Nonsteroidal anti-inflammatory drug. 70, 72, 138

Sultrin (Ob/Gyn). Topical sulfa drug for Hemophilus vaginal infection. 116, 144

Sumycin (Antibio). Tetracycline-type antibiotic.

suppository. 6, 23, 25

Suprax (Antibio). Third-generation cephalosporin antibiotic. 143

suramin (Antivir). AIDS drug. 146

Surfak (GI). Laxative. 65

Surital (Anes). Intravenous barbiturate for induction of general anesthesia. 159

Surmontil (Psych). Tricyclic antidepressant. 131

Survanta (Resp). Investigational lung surfactant supplement for premature infants. 97

Sustaire (Resp). Bronchodilator. 95

swish and swallow. 102, 148

Symmetrel (Neuro). Used to treat Parkinson disease. 122

Symmetrel (Antivir). For influenza virus A. 122, 148

Synalar (Derm). Topical corticosteroid anti-inflammatory drug. 53

Synalgos (Analges). Non-narcotic analgesic drug. 137

Synarel (Ob/Gyn). Used to treat endometriosis. 112

synergism. 37

Synkayvite (Hem). Used to reverse oral anticoagulants; also prophylactic to prevent bleeding. 93

Synthroid (Endo). Thyroid hormone replacement. 107

syrup, cough. 10, 22

syrup of ipecac (GI). To induce vomiting. 68

systemic drug effect. 32-33

■

T, t

tablet. 21, 12
  effervescent. 21
  enteric-coated. 21, 70
  scored, 21
  slow-release. 21
TACE (Ob/Gyn). Estrogen replacement for menopause. 114
tacrine (Cognex) (Neuro). Investigational drug for Alzheimer disease. 125
Tagamet (GI). H_2 blocker to heal ulcers. 6, 19, 62-63
talbutal (Lotusate) (Sed/Hyp). Barbiturate drug for insomnia. 124
Talwin (Analges). Narcotic analgesic drug. 135
Tambocor (Cardio). Antiarrhythmic drug. 79
tamoxifen (Nolvadex) (Chemo). Hormonal chemotherapy drug. 153
Tao (Antibio). Antibiotic. 145
Tapazole (Endo). Used to treat hyperthyroidism. 107
Taractan (Psych). Antipsychotic drug. 129
target organ. 33
Tavist (ENT). Decongestant. 14, 99
Tazidime (Antibio). Third-generation cephalosporin antibiotic. 143
TB (tuberculin) syringe. 43
Tedral (Resp). Bronchodilator and sedative combination drug. 95
Tegison (Derm). Oral drug for severe psoriasis. 52
Tegopen (Antibio). Penicillin-type antibiotic. 141
Tegretol (Neuro). Used to treat tonic-clonic seizures. 121
Tegrin (Derm). Coal tar shampoo/lotion for psoriasis. 52
temazepam (Restoril) (Sed/Hyp). Nonbarbiturate benzodiazepine drug for insomnia. 124
Tembid. Part of the trade name of a drug, indicating sustained-release tablet. 43
Tempra (Analges). Nonaspirin analgesic drug. 137

Tenex (Cardio). Antihypertensive drug. 83
Tenoretic (Cardio). Antihypertensive and diuretic combination drug. 84
Tenormin (Cardio, Analges). Cardioselective beta blocker drug used for angina and hypertension; also used for migraine headaches. 77, 79, 81, 138
Terazol (Ob/Gyn). Topical antiyeast drug for vaginal infections. 115
terazosin (Hytrin) (Cardio). An alpha$_1$ blocker drug for hypertension. 83
terbutaline (Brethaire, Brethine, Bricanyl) (Resp., Ob/Gyn). Bronchodilator; used to stop premature labor contractions. 95, 112
terconazole (Terazol) (Ob/Gyn). Topical antiyeast drug for vaginal infection. 115
terfenadine (Seldane) (ENT). Antihistamine. 15, 99
Terfonyl (Antibio). Sulfonamide anti-infective drug. 15, 99
terpin hydrate (ENT). Expectorant. 99
Terramycin (Antibio, Derm). Oral and topical tetracycline-type antibiotic. 53, 144
Teslac (Chemo). Hormonal chemotherapy drug. 153
Tessalon Perles (ENT). Respiratory anesthetic for intractable dry cough. 102
testing
  drug. 17-29
  in vitro drug. 17
  in vivo drug. 17
testolactone (Teslac) (Chemo). Hormonal chemotherapy drug. 153
tetracaine (Pontocaine) (Anes). Spinal/epidural anesthetic. 159
tetracaine (Pontocaine) (Derm, Oph). Topical and ophthalmic anesthetic drug. 104, 158
tetracyclic antidepressants (Psych). Class of drugs for depression. 131
tetracycline (Achromycin) (Derm, Oph). Topical and ophthalmic antibiotic. 53, 103, 117

tetracycline (Topicycline) (Derm). Topical antibiotic for acne. 51

tetracycline (Achromycin, Sumycin) (Antibio). Oral and topical antibiotic. 24, 37, 53, 116, 144

tetrahydrocannabinol (Dronabinol) (Chemo, GI). Prevents vomiting after chemotherapy. 67

thalidomide. 9

THC (GI). Abbreviation of an active ingredient in dronabinol. See *dronabinol*. 67

Theobid (Resp). Bronchodilator. 95

Theo-Dur Sprinkle (Resp). Bronchodilator. 95

Theolair (Resp). Bronchodilator. 95

Theophyl (Resp). Bronchodilator. 95

theophylline (Elixophyllin, Slo-Phyllin) (Resp). Bronchodilator. 95

Theo-24 (Resp). Bronchodilator. 95

Theovent (Resp). Bronchodilator. 95

therapeutic drug effect. 18, 32-34

therapeutic index (TI). 18, 20, 34, 43

thiamylal (Surital) (Anes). Intravenous barbiturate for induction of general anesthesia. 159

thiazide diuretics (Uro). Class of diuretic drugs. 57

thiethylperazine (Torecan) (GI). Antiemetic. 66

thioguanine (Chemo). Purine antagonist chemotherapy drug. 151

thiopental (Pentothal) (Anes). Intravenous barbiturate for induction of general anesthesia. 157, 159

thioridazine (Mellaril) (Psych). Phenothiazine antipsychotic drug. 129

Thiosulfil Forte (Uro). Sulfonamide anti-infective drug. 59, 140

thiotepa (Chemo). Alkylating chemotherapy drug. 152

thiothixene (Navane) (Psych). Antipsychotic drug. 129

Thorazine (Psych, GI). Phenothiazine antipsychotic drug; antiemetic. 6, 66-67, 128-129

thrombolytic enzymes. 92

thrush. 102, 148

thyroglobulin (Proloid) (Endo). Thyroid hormone replacement. 107

thyroid drugs. 107

Thyrolar (Endo). Thyroid hormone replacement. 107

TI (therapeutic index). 18, 20, 34, 43

Ticar (Antibio). Penicillin-type antibiotic. 141

ticarcillin (Ticar) (Antibio). Penicillin-type antibiotic. 141

Ticlid (Hem). Investigational anticoagulant. 92

ticlopidine (Ticlid) (Hem). Investigational anticoagulant. 92

t.i.d. (three times a day).

Tigan (GI). Antiemetic. 66-67

tioconazole (Vagistat) (Ob/Gyn). Topical antiyeast drug for vaginal infection. 115

Tilade (Resp). Investigational mast cell inhibitor. 96

Timentin (Antibio). Ticarcillin and beta lactamase inhibitor combination drug. 145

Timolide (Cardio). Antihypertensive and diuretic combination drug. 84

timolol (Blocadren) (Cardio, Analges). Nonselective beta blocking drug used to treat hypertension; also used for migraine headaches. 77, 79-80, 139

timolol (Timoptic) (Oph). Beta blocking drug for glaucoma. 105

Timoptic (Oph). Beta blocking drug for glaucoma. 25, 105

Tinactin (Derm). Topical antifungal drug. 54

tincture. 22

Tindal (Psych). Phenothiazine antipsychotic drug. 129

tioconazole (Vagistat) (Ob/Gyn). Topical antifungal/antiyeast drug for vaginal infection. 115

Titradose. Part of trade name of drug, indicating a scored, dividable tablet. 43

Titralac (GI). Antacid. 62

titrate the drug dose. 43

TMP (trimethoprim) (Antibio). 144

tobramycin (Nebcin) (Antibio). Aminoglycoside antibiotic. 144

tobramycin (Tobrex) (Oph). Topical antibiotic for eye. 103

Tridil (Cardio). Antianginal drug. 77

Tridione (Neuro). Used to treat absence seizures. 121

trifluoperazine (Stelazine) (Psych). Phenothiazine antipsychotic drug. 129

triflupromazine (Vesprin) (Psych, GI). Phenothiazine antipsychotic; antiemetic. 66, 129

trifluridine (Viroptic) (Oph). Topical antiviral drug for eye. 104

Trigesic (Analges). Non-narcotic analgesic drug. 137

trihexyphenidyl (Artane) (Neuro). Used to treat Parkinson disease. 123

Trilafon (Psych, GI). Phenothiazine antipsychotic drug; antiemetic. 66-67, 129

Tri-Levlen (Ob/Gyn). Combination triphasic progesterone/estrogen oral contraceptive. 113

Trilisate (Ortho). Nonsteroidal anti-inflammatory drug. 70, 136

trimethadione (Tridione) (Neuro). Used to treat absence seizures. 121

trimethobenzamide (Tigan) (GI). Antiemetic. 66-67

trimethoprim (TMP) (Antibio). 144

trimipramine (Surmontil) (Psych). Tricyclic antidepressant. 131

Trimox (Antibio). Penicillin-type antibiotic. 141

Trinalin (ENT). Decongestant and antihistamine combination drug. 100

Tri-Norinyl (Ob/Gyn). Combination triphasic progesterone/estrogen oral contraceptive. 113

Trinsicon. Oral vitamin B_{12} with iron and vitamin C. 87

triphasic oral contraceptives (Ob/Gyn). Class of drugs for oral contraception using three different levels of progesterone per month. 113

Triphasil (Ob/Gyn). Combination triphasic progesterone/estrogen oral contraceptive. 113

triple dye (Derm). 56

triple sulfa (Sultrin) (Ob/Gyn). Topical sulfa drug for *Hemophilus* vaginal infection. 116

triple sulfa (Terfonyl) (Uro). Oral sulfonamide anti-infective. 59, 140

Triple X (Derm). Topical drug for pediculosis or lice. 55

Trobicin (Antibio). Oral antibiotic. 117

troche. 102, 148

troleandomycin (Tao) (Antibio). Antibiotic. 145

Tronothane (Derm). Topical anesthetic. 158

tropicamide (Ophth). Mydriatic drug. 105

trough level of drug. 43

tuberculin (TB) syringe. 43

tuberculosis, drugs for. 96

tubocurarine (Anes). Intraoperative muscle-paralyzing drug. 160

Tuinal (Sed/Hyp). Combination of two barbiturates. 125

Tums (GI). Antacid. 62

Tussi-Organidin (ENT). Expectorant and narcotic antitussive combination drug. 10, 100

Tylenol (Analges). Non-narcotic non-aspirin analgesic drug. 21-23, 25, 70, 137

Tylenol With Codeine (Analges). Narcotic analgesic drug. 10, 37, 137

Tylenol With Codeine No. 1 (Analges). Tylenol with 7.5 mg codeine. 137

Tylenol With Codeine No. 2 (Analges). Tylenol with 15 mg codeine. 137

Tylenol With Codeine No. 3 (Analges). Tylenol with 30 mg codeine. 137

Tylenol With Codeine No. 4 (Analges). Tylenol with 60 mg codeine. 137

■

U, u

U-100 (Endo). 100 units of insulin per milliliter. 45

Uendex (Antivir). AIDS drug. 146

ulcer, drugs for. 61-63

ulcerative colitis, drugs for. 65-66

Ultracef (Antibio). First-generation cephalosporin antibiotic. 143

Ultradol (Ortho). Investigational nonsteroidal anti-inflammatory drug. 70, 138

Ultralente Iletin (Endo). Injectable ultralente insulin. 109

ultralente insulin (Humulin U) (Endo). Injectable ultralente insulin. 109

Unasyn (Antibio). Ampicillin and beta lactamase inhibitor combination drug. 145

Unicard (Cardio). Investigative nonselective beta blocking drug. 80

Unipen (Antibio). Penicillin-type antibiotic. 141

Unisom (Sed./Hyp). Over-the-counter non-barbiturate drug for insomnia. 124

unit, insulin. 45

Unit, International (IU). 45

United States Adopted Names Council. 13

United States Pharmacopeia. 8

uracil mustard (Chemo). Alkylating chemotherapy drug. 152

Urecholine (Uro). Urinary antispasmodic drug. 60

urinary tract, drugs for. 57-60

Urispas (Uro). Antispasmodic. 59

urofollitropin (Metrodin) (Ob/Gyn). Ovulation-stimulating drug for infertility. 111

Urogesic (Uro). Urinary tract analgesic. 59

urokinase (Abbokinase) (Cardio, Hem). Thrombolytic enzyme. 92

ursodiol (Actigall) (GI). Used to dissolve gallstones. 68

uterine relaxants. 112

uterine stimulants. 112

Uticort (Derm). Topical corticosteroid anti-inflammatory drug. 53

Utimox (Antibio). Penicillin-type antibiotic. 141

V, v

vaginal drug administration. 25, 28

vaginal infections, drugs for. 115-116

Vagistat (Ob/Gyn). Topical antiyeast drug for vaginal infections. 115

Valisone (Derm). Topical corticosteroid anti-inflammatory drug. 53

Valium (Psych, Neuro). Benzodiazepine antianxiety drug; also used for status epilepticus. 13, 15, 125, 127

Valium (Anes). Preoperative drug to decrease anxiety, provide sedation. 160

Valium (Ortho). Skeletal muscle relaxant. 72

Valmid (Sed/Hyp). Nonbarbiturate drug for insomnia. 123

Valpin (GI). Antispasmodic drug. 64

valproic acid (Depakene) (Neuro). Used to treat absence seizures. 121

Vancenase (ENT). Intranasal corticosteroid. 101

Vanceril (Resp). Corticosteroid. 95

Vancocin (Antibio). Antibiotic. 145

vancomycin (Vancocin) (Antibio). Antibiotic. 145

van Gogh, Vincent. 76

Vanquish (Analges). Non-narcotic analgesic drug. 137

Vaseretic (Cardio). Antihypertensive and diuretic combination drug. 84

Vasodilan (Cardio). Peripheral vasodilating drug. 84

vasodilators (Cardio). Class of drugs which dilate blood vessels. 43, 83-84

vasopressin (Pitressin) (Endo). Used to treat diabetes insipidus. 108

vasopressors (Cardio). Class of drugs which constrict blood vessels and raise blood pressure. 90

Vasotec (Cardio). ACE inhibitor drug used for hypertension. 82

Vasoxyl (Anes). Used to treat hypotension from spinal anesthesia. 161

Vasotec (Cardio). ACE inhibitor drug used for hypertension. 82

Vasoxyl (Anes). Used to treat hypotension from spinal anesthesia. 161

V-Cillin K (Antibio). Penicillin-type antibiotic. 116-117, 141

vecuronium (Norcuron) (Anes). Intraoperative muscle-paralyzing drug. 160

Velban (Chemo). Mitotic inhibiting chemotherapy drug. 153

Velosef (Antibio). Cephalosporin antibiotic. 35

Velosulin (Endo). Injectable regular insulin. 109

Ventolin (Resp). Bronchodilator. 94

VePesid (Chemo). Mitotic inhibiting chemotherapy drug. 153

verapamil (Calan, Isoptin) (Cardio, Analges). Calcium channel blocker drug for angina, arrhythmias, and hypertension; also for migraine headaches. 6, 78-79, 82, 139

Vercyte (Chemo). Alkylating chemotherapy drug. 152

Verelan (Cardio, Analges). Calcium channel blocking drug for angina, arrhythmias, and hypertension; also for migraine headaches. 78, 82

Versed (Anes). Intravenous drug for induction of general anesthesia. 159

Vesprin (Psych, GI) Phenothiazine antipsychotic drug; antiemetic. 66, 129

vial. 43

Vibramycin (Antibio). Tetracycline-type antibiotic. 116-117, 144

Vicodin (Analges). Narcotic analgesic. 137

vidarabine (Ara-A, Vira-A) (Antivir). Injectable drug for herpes simplex virus. 148

vidarabine (Vira-A) (Oph). Topical antiviral drug. 104

vinblastine (Velban) (Chemo). Mitotic inhibiting chemotherapy drug. 153

vinca (plant). 5, 153

vincristine (Oncovin) (Chemo). Mitotic inhibiting chemotherapy drug. 5, 153

vindesine (Eldisine) (Chemo). Investigative mitotic inhibiting chemotherapy drug. 153